POLYMYALGIA RHEUMATICA

DIET COOKBOOK

FOR BEGINNERS

Simple, Nourishing Recipes to Alleviate Pain, Reduce Inflammation, and Boost Energy Levels

Kingsley Klopp

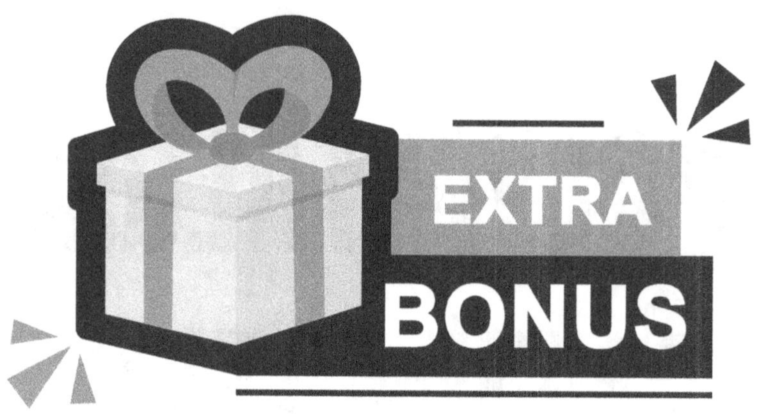

To show our appreciation for your purchase, we're delighted to offer you these special bonuses as a heartfelt thank you.

1. A Food Tracker Journal
2. Downloadable E-BOOK featuring full-color images of finished recipes

Table of Contents

Snacks & Sides Recipes

Desserts Recipes

Important Note

Polymyalgia Rheumatica affects each individual differently, and while this cookbook offers a variety of recipes designed to support your health, it's essential to remember that everyone's dietary needs are unique. What works wonderfully for one person might not be the perfect fit for another. Therefore, we encourage you to listen to your body and make adjustments to the recipes as needed to best suit your personal health requirements.

We've provided approximate nutritional information for each recipe to guide you in making informed choices. However, keep in mind that these values may vary based on the specific brands and types of ingredients you use. For example, the size of a vegetable or the brand of a product can influence the nutritional content. We recommend using this information as a general guide and not an absolute measurement.

As you experiment with these recipes, it's crucial to consult with your healthcare provider, especially if you're uncertain about any dietary changes. Your doctor or a registered dietitian can offer personalized advice tailored to your specific health needs and conditions. They can help you understand which foods are best for managing your symptoms and overall well-being.

Our goal is to empower you with delicious, nutritious options that can help alleviate the symptoms of Polymyalgia Rheumatica and improve your quality of life. We hope you find joy and comfort in the process of preparing and enjoying these meals, knowing that each bite is a step towards better health.

Furthermore, If our cookbook has brought joy to your kitchen and table, we'd be thrilled to hear about your experiences in an Amazon review. On the flip side, if you stumble upon any hiccups while exploring our recipes, don't hesitate to get in touch at **kloppkingsley@gmail.com.** We're here to support your cooking journey every step of the way.

Happy cooking, and here's to your health and happiness!

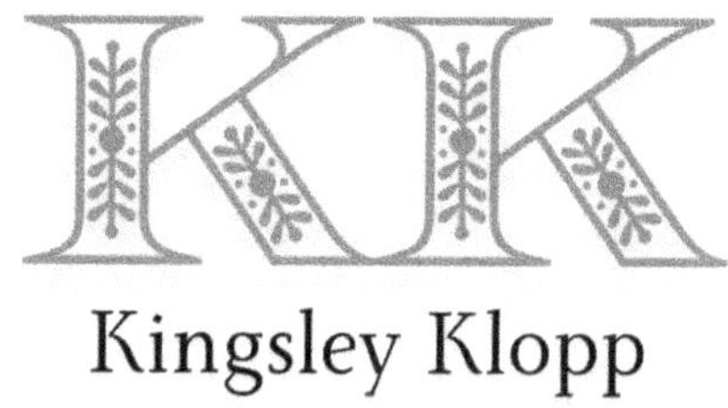

Kingsley Klopp

Introduction.

Welcome to the **Polymyalgia Rheumatica Diet Cookbook for Beginners**! If you're here, it's likely because either you or someone close to you is navigating the challenging path of living with Polymyalgia Rheumatica (PMR). Whether you've been recently diagnosed or have been living with PMR for some time, you're about to embark on a journey that will empower you to take control of your health and well-being through the power of nutrition. Polymyalgia Rheumatica can feel like an uninvited guest in your life, bringing with it pain, stiffness, and fatigue that can overshadow even the simplest daily activities. It's a condition that often leaves you feeling frustrated and helpless, searching for ways to alleviate the symptoms and improve your quality of life. But here's the good news: you've already taken the first crucial step towards managing PMR by seeking out dietary solutions. And that's exactly where this cookbook comes in. In these pages, you'll find more than just recipes. You'll discover a comprehensive guide that combines the latest nutritional science with practical, easy-to-follow meal plans designed specifically for those with PMR. We'll explore the connection between diet and inflammation, uncovering how certain foods can either exacerbate or help manage your symptoms. Imagine having the knowledge and tools at your fingertips to make informed food choices that could potentially reduce your pain and stiffness, boost your energy levels, and improve your overall health.

But let's be real: adopting a new diet can be daunting. It can feel overwhelming to sift through endless information, trying to figure out what's best for you. That's why this cookbook is tailored for beginners. We're starting from scratch, breaking down the essentials of a PMR-friendly diet in a way that's straightforward and accessible. You don't need to be a culinary expert or a nutritionist to benefit from this book; all you need is a willingness to learn and a desire to feel better. You might be wondering, "What can I expect from this cookbook?" Well, get ready for a diverse array of delicious, nutrient-packed recipes that cater to a variety of tastes and dietary preferences. From hearty breakfasts to sustain you through the morning, to satisfying dinners that bring comfort after a long day, we've got you covered. Each recipe is crafted with anti-inflammatory ingredients that are both easy to find and simple to prepare. We've also included tips and tricks for meal planning, shopping lists, and even suggestions for dining out, so you'll feel confident and prepared in any situation.

However, the focus of this book is on cultivating a lifestyle that promotes your health and wellbeing, not only eating. We'll discuss the importance of hydration, the role of physical activity, and how stress management can play a part in managing PMR. Consider this cookbook your companion on a journey towards a more vibrant, energetic, and pain-free life.

So, let's get started. Turn the page and dive into a world where delicious food meets healthful living. Together, we'll explore the flavors, textures, and benefits of a diet designed to help you thrive despite Polymyalgia Rheumatica. Welcome to your new culinary adventure, where each meal is a step towards a healthier, happier you.

Chapter 1: Understanding Polymyalgia Rheumatica

What is Polymyalgia Rheumatica?.

Polymyalgia Rheumatica (PMR) is a condition that quietly creeps into the lives of those affected, often leaving them in a state of confusion and despair. Imagine waking up one morning, unable to lift your arms to brush your hair, or struggling to get out of bed because your hips and shoulders are so stiff and painful. This is the reality for many people living with PMR, a chronic inflammatory disorder that primarily affects older adults.PMR is not just a medical term; it is a thief of joy and mobility. The name itself translates to "pain in many muscles," and it is an apt description. The pain and stiffness are not localized to one area but are widespread, typically affecting the shoulders, neck, arms, and hips. These symptoms can be severe, making it difficult for individuals to perform even the simplest of daily tasks. Dressing, bathing, and cooking can become monumental challenges, stripping away the independence that many have enjoyed throughout their lives. The onset of PMR can be sudden and striking. One day, an individual may feel perfectly fine, and the next, they are grappling with debilitating pain and stiffness. This rapid change can be frightening and bewildering, leading to a significant emotional toll. The unpredictability of PMR means that patients often live in fear of when the next flare-up will occur, constantly on edge and anxious about their condition.

Diagnosing PMR can be a complex process, adding another layer of frustration for those affected. There is no specific test for PMR; instead, doctors must rely on a combination of symptoms, physical examination, and blood tests to arrive at a diagnosis. These blood tests typically look for elevated levels of inflammatory markers, such as erythrocyte sedimentation rate (ESR) and C-reactive protein (CRP). However, these markers are not unique to PMR, making the diagnostic journey a lengthy and often discouraging one. Patients may see multiple specialists, undergo numerous tests, and still feel no closer to an answer. Once diagnosed, the primary treatment for PMR is corticosteroids, such as prednisone. These medications can work wonders in reducing inflammation and alleviating symptoms, often bringing significant relief within days. However, they are not without their downsides. Long-term use of corticosteroids can lead to a host of side effects, including weight gain, high blood pressure, diabetes, and osteoporosis. Patients are faced with a difficult choice: endure the debilitating symptoms of PMR or risk the potential complications of long-term steroid use.

Living with PMR is a daily battle. The physical pain and stiffness are constant reminders of the condition, but the emotional impact is equally profound. Many individuals with PMR feel a sense of isolation and depression, as their condition limits their ability to participate in social activities and hobbies they once loved. The fear of being perceived as a burden on family and friends can lead to a sense of guilt and worthlessness. It is not uncommon for those with PMR to experience a grieving process, mourning the loss of their former, more active selves. Despite these challenges, there is hope for those living with PMR. Support from family, friends, and healthcare providers is crucial in managing the condition. Physical therapy and gentle exercise can help maintain mobility and strength, while support groups provide a space for individuals to share their experiences and connect with others who understand their struggles. Advances in medical research continue to shed light on PMR, bringing us closer to more effective treatments and potentially even a cure.

Hence, Polymyalgia Rheumatica is more than just a medical condition; it is a life-altering experience that affects every aspect of a person's life. The physical pain and stiffness are only part of the story; the emotional and psychological impact is just as significant. Understanding PMR means recognizing the courage and resilience of those who live with it every day. It is a reminder that behind every diagnosis is a human being, facing their battles with strength and determination. PMR may steal moments of joy and mobility, but it cannot take away the spirit of those who continue to fight against it.

Symptoms and Diagnosis of Polymyalgia Rheumatica

Symptoms of Polymyalgia Rheumatica

The hallmark symptoms of PMR are muscle pain and stiffness, particularly in the shoulders, neck, and hips. These symptoms can develop suddenly, over a few days, or gradually over a longer period. They are typically more pronounced in the morning or after periods of inactivity, making it difficult for individuals to get out of bed or move around after sitting for a while.

1. **Pain and Stiffness**:
   - The pain is usually bilateral, affecting both sides of the body. It can be severe, throbbing, and deep-seated.
   - Stiffness is most intense in the morning and can last for more than an hour, significantly reducing mobility and flexibility.
2. **Fatigue**:
   - People with PMR often experience overwhelming fatigue. This can make it challenging to carry out daily tasks and can contribute to a general feeling of malaise.
3. **Fever and Weight Loss**:
   - Low-grade fever and unexplained weight loss can also be symptoms of PMR. These signs can be subtle but are important indicators of the systemic inflammation characteristic of the condition.
4. **Decreased Appetite**:
   - Many people with PMR report a reduced appetite, which can lead to nutritional deficiencies and further exacerbate fatigue and weight loss.
5. **Depression and Mood Changes**:
   - Chronic pain and fatigue can lead to depression and anxiety. The inability to participate in previously enjoyed activities can take a toll on mental health.
6. **Swelling and Tenderness**:
   - In some cases, swelling and tenderness may occur in the wrists, knees, and small joints of the hands and feet.

Diagnosis of Polymyalgia Rheumatica

Diagnosing PMR can be a complex process, as its symptoms often overlap with those of other conditions, such as rheumatoid arthritis, lupus, and fibromyalgia. There is no single test for PMR; instead, the diagnosis is based on a combination of clinical evaluation, patient history, and laboratory tests.

1. **Clinical Evaluation**:
   - A thorough physical examination is conducted to assess pain, stiffness, and swelling. The doctor will also review the patient's medical history and symptom onset to identify patterns that are characteristic of PMR.

2. **Laboratory Tests**:
    - **Erythrocyte Sedimentation Rate (ESR)**: This test measures the rate at which red blood cells settle at the bottom of a test tube. A high ESR indicates inflammation in the body.
    - **C-reactive Protein (CRP)**: This protein is produced by the liver in response to inflammation. Elevated levels of CRP are common in PMR.
    - **Complete Blood Count (CBC)**: This test can help rule out other conditions by providing a comprehensive overview of the patient's overall health.
3. **Response to Treatment**:
    - One of the defining characteristics of PMR is its rapid response to corticosteroids, such as prednisone. If symptoms improve dramatically within a few days of starting treatment, it supports the diagnosis of PMR.
4. **Exclusion of Other Conditions**:
    - The doctor will work to exclude other conditions with similar symptoms. This might involve additional tests, such as imaging studies (X-rays, ultrasound, or MRI) to check for joint and tissue abnormalities or to rule out other forms of arthritis.

Challenges in Diagnosis

The diagnostic process can be frustrating for patients due to the nonspecific nature of PMR symptoms and the need to rule out other conditions. Additionally, older adults often have multiple health issues that can obscure the diagnosis. It's important for patients to communicate clearly with their healthcare providers about all symptoms and any changes in their condition.

Treatment Options for Polymyalgia Rheumatica

Polymyalgia Rheumatica (PMR) is a chronic inflammatory disorder that causes widespread muscle pain and stiffness, particularly in the shoulders, neck, and hips. While the symptoms can be debilitating, effective treatment options are available that can help manage the condition and improve the quality of life for those affected. The primary goal of treatment is to reduce inflammation, alleviate pain, and maintain mobility.

1. Corticosteroids

Corticosteroids are the cornerstone of PMR treatment. Prednisone, a type of corticosteroid, is typically prescribed at the onset of the disease.

- **Prednisone:** Most patients experience significant relief from symptoms within a few days of starting prednisone. The initial dose is usually moderate, and once symptoms are controlled, the dosage is gradually reduced to the lowest effective level. The duration of corticosteroid therapy can range from six months to two years or longer, depending on the individual's response to treatment and the presence of any relapses.
- **Side Effects:** Long-term use of corticosteroids can lead to side effects such as weight gain, high blood pressure, diabetes, osteoporosis, and increased risk of infections. Therefore, it is important to monitor patients closely and manage these potential complications.

2. Nonsteroidal Anti-Inflammatory Drugs (NSAIDs)

NSAIDs, such as ibuprofen and naproxen, can be used to relieve mild to moderate pain and inflammation.

- **Use in PMR:** While NSAIDs may provide some symptom relief, they are generally not as effective as corticosteroids for controlling the underlying inflammation of PMR. They are often used as adjunct therapy in combination with corticosteroids.
- **Side Effects:** NSAIDs can cause gastrointestinal issues, including stomach ulcers and bleeding, especially with long-term use. They can also affect kidney function and increase the risk of cardiovascular problems.

3. Disease-Modifying Antirheumatic Drugs (DMARDs)

In some cases, particularly when patients cannot tolerate corticosteroids or require long-term treatment at higher doses, DMARDs may be considered.

- **Methotrexate:** This is one of the most commonly used DMARDs in PMR. It can help reduce the need for corticosteroids and manage symptoms effectively.
- **Other DMARDs:** Leflunomide and hydroxychloroquine are other options that might be considered, although their use in PMR is less common.

4. Lifestyle Modifications

Lifestyle changes play a significant role in managing PMR and minimizing the side effects of treatment.

- **Diet**: A balanced diet rich in fruits, vegetables, whole grains, and lean proteins can help maintain overall health. Calcium and vitamin D supplements may be recommended to protect bone health, especially in patients taking corticosteroids.
- **Exercise**: Gentle exercise, such as walking, swimming, or yoga, can help maintain mobility and reduce stiffness. Physical therapy may also be beneficial in designing an appropriate exercise program tailored to the individual's needs.
- **Stress Management**: Chronic pain and illness can lead to stress and emotional distress. Techniques such as meditation, deep breathing exercises, and mindfulness can help manage stress levels and improve mental well-being.

5. Monitoring and Follow-Up

Regular monitoring and follow-up with a healthcare provider are essential to ensure effective management of PMR and to adjust treatment as needed.

- **Blood Tests**: Regular blood tests to monitor inflammatory markers (ESR and CRP) help assess the effectiveness of treatment and detect any flares or relapses.
- **Bone Health**: Monitoring bone density is important, especially for patients on long-term corticosteroid therapy, to prevent osteoporosis and fractures.

6. Emerging Therapies

Research into new treatment options for PMR is ongoing, and emerging therapies may offer additional options in the future.

- **Biologic Agents**: These drugs, which target specific components of the immune system, are being studied for their potential use in PMR. Tocilizumab, an IL-6 receptor antagonist, has shown promise in some studies.
- **New Corticosteroid Formulations**: Researchers are exploring alternative formulations and delivery methods for corticosteroids that may reduce side effects and improve patient outcomes.

Nutritional Needs and Considerations

When grappling with Polymyalgia Rheumatica (PMR), the body demands more than just medical treatment—it seeks nourishment that can soothe inflammation, strengthen bones, and replenish energy. Understanding the nutritional needs and adapting your diet accordingly can transform the way you live with PMR. It's not merely about eating; it's about feeding the soul, comforting the body, and fostering a sense of well-being through the healing power of food.

Fueling the Fight Against Inflammation

The central battle in PMR is against inflammation. Adjusting your diet to include anti-inflammatory foods can significantly influence how you feel. Foods rich in omega-3 fatty acids, such as salmon, flaxseeds, and walnuts, are known for their anti-inflammatory properties. Integrating these into your daily meals can help reduce inflammation levels and alleviate some of the stiffness and pain associated with PMR.

Similarly, fruits and vegetables are not just sides to your meals; they are your allies. Berries, leafy greens, and other brightly colored fruits and vegetables are loaded with antioxidants and phytochemicals that combat inflammation. Imagine starting your day with a smoothie that not only tastes good but also reduces your body's inflammatory response.

Supporting Bone Health

Corticosteroids, often prescribed for PMR, can lead to decreased bone density and increased risk of osteoporosis. Therefore, it is crucial to include calcium-rich foods to support bone health. Dairy products, fortified plant milks, and green leafy vegetables are excellent sources of calcium. Pair these with vitamin D-rich foods like fatty fish and fortified cereals, or consider a vitamin D supplement, to enhance calcium absorption and bone strength. This combination doesn't just protect your bones; it builds a fortress around them, enhancing your resilience against the potential side effects of long-term steroid use.

Managing Weight and Blood Sugar

Steroids can also affect your weight and blood sugar levels, adding an emotional burden to an already challenging situation. Managing your diet to prevent weight gain and stabilize blood sugar becomes essential. Focus on whole grains, lean proteins, and fiber-rich foods which help in slowing down sugar absorption and maintaining a healthy weight. Imagine your plate as a palette of colors, filled with a variety of foods that keep your body nourished, your blood sugar stable, and your weight under control.

Spices: The Natural Healers

Embrace the power of spices in your diet. Turmeric, for instance, contains curcumin, a compound with potent anti-inflammatory properties. Adding a teaspoon of turmeric to your meals can help reduce inflammation naturally. Ginger and garlic also offer similar benefits, adding flavor and a therapeutic touch to your dishes.

Hydration: The Essence of Vitality

Hydration plays a pivotal role in managing PMR. Water helps flush out toxins, aids in digestion, and keeps your joints lubricated. It's not just about quenching thirst; it's about ensuring that every cell in your body works optimally, reducing the risk of flare-ups.

Foods to Include in a Polymyalgia Rheumatica Diet

When managing a condition like Polymyalgia Rheumatica (PMR), each meal plays a crucial role not just in nourishing the body, but also in combating the inflammation that characterizes this condition. Including the right foods in your diet can significantly alleviate symptoms, enhance your energy levels, and improve your overall quality of life. Here's a closer look at the types of foods that should be staples in your diet if you're battling PMR.

Rich in Omega-3 Fatty Acids

Foods high in omega-3 fatty acids are essential for their anti-inflammatory properties. These nutrients can help reduce the cytokine levels in the body, which are substances that promote inflammation. Include these foods regularly:

- **Fatty Fish:** Salmon, mackerel, sardines, and trout are excellent sources of marine omega-3s which are particularly effective against inflammation.
- **Flaxseeds and Chia Seeds:** These seeds are not only high in omega-3s but also fiber, which can help improve your digestive health.
- **Walnuts:** Perfect as a snack or as an addition to salads, walnuts are a versatile source of omega-3s.

Antioxidant-Rich Fruits and Vegetables

Antioxidants play a critical role in neutralizing free radicals in the body, which can contribute to inflammation and cell damage. Incorporating a variety of colorful fruits and vegetables ensures a broad spectrum of antioxidants and nutrients:

- **Berries:** Strawberries, blueberries, and blackberries are rich in vitamins and antioxidants.
- **Leafy Greens:** Spinach, kale, and Swiss chard contain high levels of vitamins and minerals, along with anti-inflammatory properties.
- **Cruciferous Vegetables:** Broccoli, cauliflower, and Brussels sprouts are known for their health benefits, including their potential to fight inflammation.

Whole Grains

Whole grains are packed with fiber, which helps in managing weight and reducing the impact of high blood sugar levels that can be a side effect of steroid treatment:

- **Oats:** Great for breakfast, oats can help maintain a steady blood sugar level.
- **Quinoa and Brown Rice:** These grains are excellent bases for meals, adding substance and nutrition without exacerbating inflammation.

Lean Proteins

Maintaining muscle mass is crucial, especially in seniors dealing with PMR. Lean proteins can help in muscle repair and maintenance without contributing to inflammation:

- **Chicken and Turkey Breast:** Opt for skinless options to reduce fat intake.
- **Legumes:** Beans, lentils, and chickpeas are not only high in protein but also fiber, making them excellent for digestion and heart health.

Calcium and Vitamin D Rich Foods

Since steroid use can deplete bone density, it's important to include sources of calcium and vitamin D in your diet:

- **Dairy Products:** Milk, yogurt, and cheese are traditional sources of calcium. Choose low-fat options to avoid extra saturated fat.
- **Fortified Foods:** Some plant milks and cereals are fortified with calcium and vitamin D, making them good alternatives for those who are lactose intolerant or vegan.

Healthy Fats

Healthy fats are crucial for overall health and help absorb vitamins that are fat-soluble:

- **Avocados:** Rich in monounsaturated fats and fiber, avocados are beneficial for heart health and may aid in reducing inflammation.
- **Olive Oil:** Use it in cooking or as a salad dressing base for an additional anti-inflammatory boost.

Herbs and Spices

Incorporating certain herbs and spices can add flavor without the need for salt, which should be limited in a PMR diet:

- **Turmeric:** Contains curcumin, which has strong anti-inflammatory properties.
- **Ginger:** Helps in reducing nausea and can also lower inflammation.

Foods to Avoid in a Polymyalgia Rheumatica Diet

For individuals managing Polymyalgia Rheumatica (PMR), paying attention to diet is as much about knowing what to avoid as it is about knowing what to include. Certain foods can exacerbate inflammation, leading to increased pain and stiffness. Steering clear of these can help mitigate symptoms and improve overall wellbeing. Here's a guide on which foods to limit or avoid to help manage the inflammation associated with PMR.

Processed and Red Meats
- **Why to Avoid:** Processed meats (like sausages, bacon, and deli meats) and red meats can promote inflammatory responses in the body due to their high levels of saturated fats and advanced glycation end products, substances formed when these meats are cooked at high temperatures.
- **Alternative Choices:** Opt for lean proteins such as chicken, turkey, or plant-based proteins like beans and lentils, which do not promote inflammation.

Refined Carbohydrates and Sugars
- **Why to Avoid:** White bread, pastries, and sugary snacks can cause a spike in blood sugar and insulin levels, which in turn can trigger an inflammatory response.
- **Alternative Choices:** Choose whole grains like oats, quinoa, and whole-wheat products, which help maintain steady blood sugar levels and are packed with fiber.

Fried and High-Fat Foods
- **Why to Avoid:** Foods that are fried or high in trans fats can increase inflammation and are also detrimental to heart health.
- **Alternative Choices:** Use cooking methods like baking, steaming, or grilling instead of frying, and choose heart-healthy oils like olive oil.

Dairy Products
- **Why to Avoid:** Some individuals find that dairy products can exacerbate inflammation, especially if they have a sensitivity to lactose or casein, which are found in milk and other dairy products.
- **Alternative Choices:** Experiment with lactose-free dairy products or plant-based alternatives such as almond, soy, or oat milks that are fortified with calcium and vitamin D.

Artificial Additives
- **Why to Avoid:** Artificial colorings, preservatives, and flavorings found in many processed foods can aggravate inflammation and contribute to other health issues.
- **Alternative Choices:** Focus on whole, unprocessed foods to avoid these additives naturally.

Certain Vegetables and Legumes

- **Why to Avoid:** While vegetables are generally healthy, some, like tomatoes, eggplants, and peppers, belong to the nightshade family and may trigger inflammation in some people sensitive to these types of vegetables. Similarly, some legumes like chickpeas and black beans can cause bloating and discomfort in some individuals.
- **Alternative Choices:** If you notice symptoms flare after consuming these, it might be helpful to reduce their intake and monitor your response.

Alcohol and Caffeine

- **Why to Avoid:** Alcohol can increase inflammation and interfere with the effectiveness of medications. Caffeine can disrupt sleep patterns and exacerbate stress responses, which may worsen symptoms.
- **Alternative Choices:** Limit or avoid alcohol and consider decaffeinated versions of coffee and tea.

High-Sodium Foods

- **Why to Avoid:** Excessive salt intake can lead to water retention, increased blood pressure, and strain on the kidneys, all of which can exacerbate symptoms of PMR.
- **Alternative Choices:** Limit the use of table salt and check labels for sodium content, especially in processed foods. Enhance flavor with herbs and spices instead.

Breakfast Recipes

1. Blueberry Spinach Smoothie

Ingredients:

- 1 cup fresh spinach leaves
- 1 cup frozen blueberries
- 1 medium banana
- 1 cup unsweetened almond milk
- 1 tablespoon chia seeds
- 1 teaspoon honey (optional)

Instructions:

1. Combine all ingredients in a blender.
2. Blend on high until smooth and creamy.
3. Pour into a glass and enjoy immediately.

Nutrition Info (per serving):

- Calories: 180
- Protein: 4g
- Carbohydrates: 36g
- Dietary Fiber: 8g
- Sugars: 18g
- Fat: 4g
- Saturated Fat: 0.5g
- Sodium: 150mg

Serves: 1

Cooking Time: 5 minutes

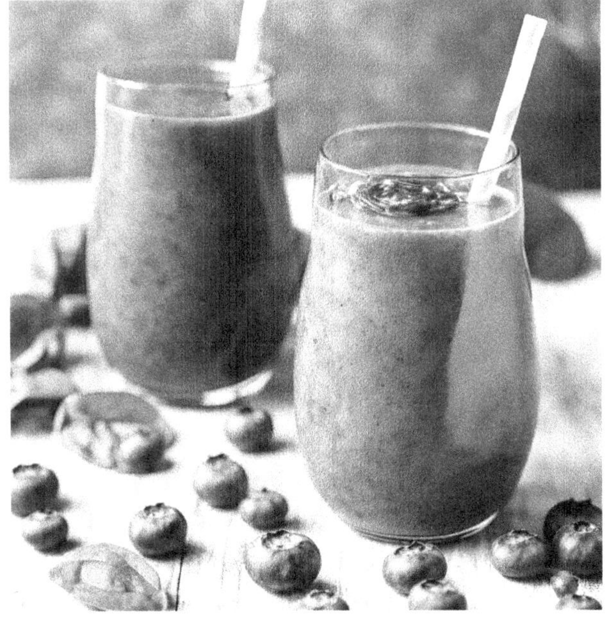

2. Cherry Almond Smoothie

Ingredients:

- 1 cup frozen cherries
- 1 medium banana
- 1 cup unsweetened almond milk
- 2 tablespoons almond butter
- 1 teaspoon vanilla extract
- 1 teaspoon maple syrup (optional)

Instructions:

1. Combine all ingredients in a blender.
2. Blend on high until smooth and creamy.
3. Pour into a glass and enjoy immediately.

Nutrition Info (per serving):

- Calories: 300
- Protein: 6g
- Carbohydrates: 41g
- Dietary Fiber: 6g
- Sugars: 24g
- Fat: 15g
- Saturated Fat: 1g
- Sodium: 170mg

Serves: 1

Cooking Time: 5 minutes

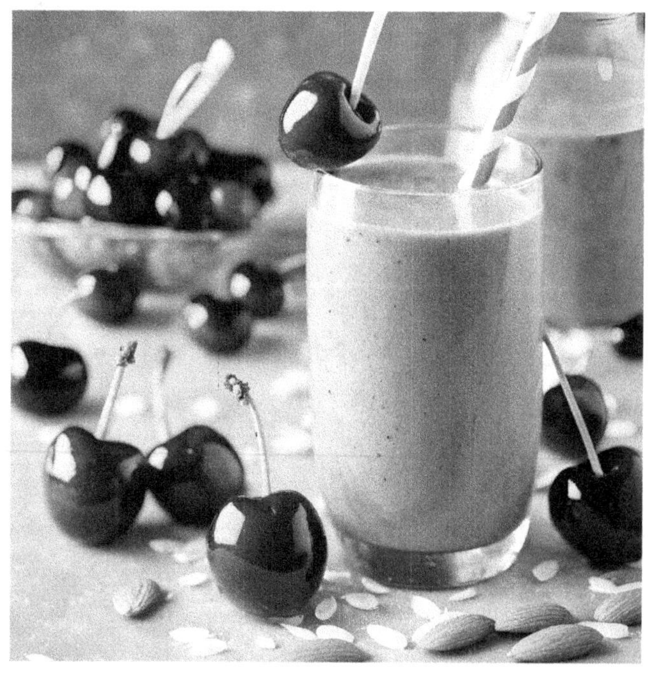

3. Oatmeal with Walnuts and Berries

Ingredients:

- 1 cup rolled oats
- 2 cups water
- 1/2 cup fresh mixed berries (blueberries, strawberries, raspberries)
- 1/4 cup chopped walnuts
- 1 tablespoon honey
- 1/2 teaspoon cinnamon

Instructions:

1. In a medium saucepan, bring water to a boil.
2. Add oats and reduce heat to medium, cooking for 5-7 minutes, stirring occasionally, until the oats are soft and the water is absorbed.
3. Remove from heat and stir in the honey and cinnamon.
4. Top with fresh berries and chopped walnuts before serving.

Nutrition Info (per serving):

- Calories: 350
- Protein: 9g
- Carbohydrates: 52g
- Dietary Fiber: 8g
- Sugars: 15g
- Fat: 14g
- Saturated Fat: 1.5g
- Sodium: 5mg

Serves: 2

Cooking Time: 10 minutes

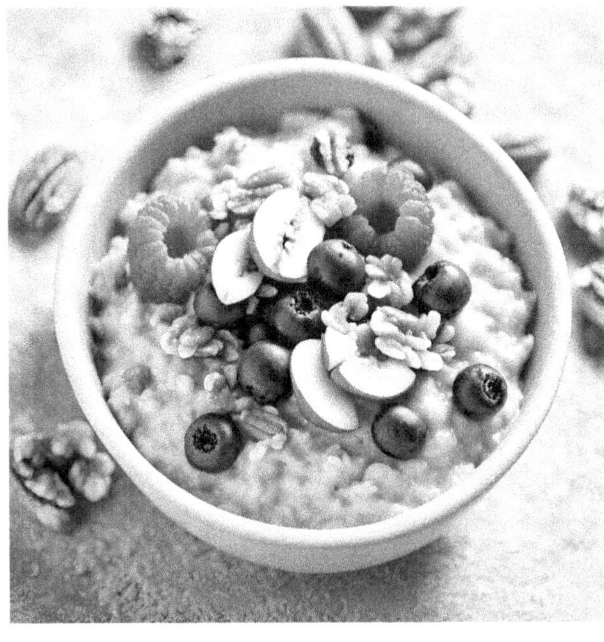

4. Quinoa Porridge

Ingredients:

- 1 cup quinoa, rinsed
- 2 cups unsweetened almond milk
- 1 tablespoon maple syrup
- 1 teaspoon vanilla extract
- 1/2 teaspoon ground cinnamon
- 1/4 cup fresh berries
- 1 tablespoon chopped almonds

Instructions:

1. In a medium saucepan, combine quinoa and almond milk. Bring to a boil over medium heat.
2. Reduce heat to low and simmer, covered, for about 15 minutes or until the quinoa is tender and the liquid is absorbed.
3. Stir in the maple syrup, vanilla extract, and cinnamon.
4. Divide into bowls and top with fresh berries and chopped almonds.

Nutrition Info (per serving):

- Calories: 280
- Protein: 8g
- Carbohydrates: 45g
- Dietary Fiber: 5g
- Sugars: 10g
- Fat: 8g
- Saturated Fat: 0.5g
- Sodium: 80mg

Serves: 2

Cooking Time: 20 minutes

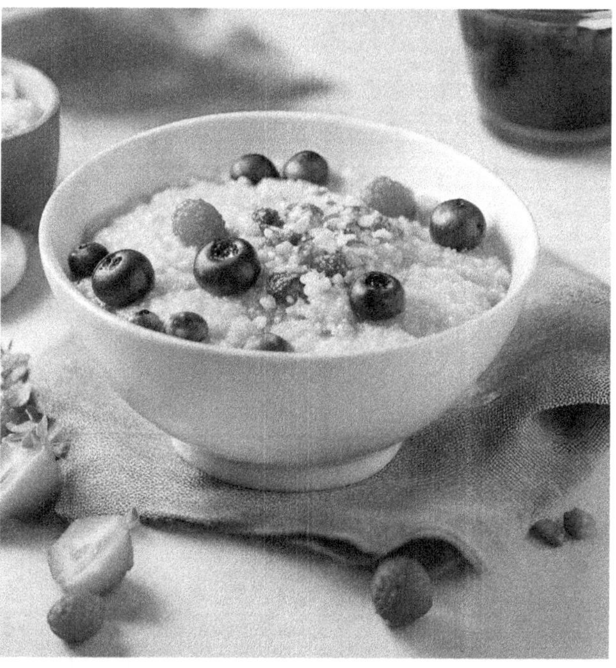

5. Turmeric Scrambled Eggs

Ingredients:

- 4 large eggs
- 1/4 cup unsweetened almond milk
- 1 teaspoon turmeric powder
- 1/4 teaspoon black pepper
- 1 tablespoon olive oil
- 1/2 cup baby spinach leaves

Instructions:

1. In a bowl, whisk together the eggs, almond milk, turmeric, and black pepper.
2. Heat olive oil in a non-stick skillet over medium heat.
3. Add the spinach and cook until wilted, about 1-2 minutes.
4. Pour in the egg mixture and cook, stirring frequently, until the eggs are fully cooked and scrambled, about 3-4 minutes.
5. Serve immediately.

Nutrition Info (per serving):

- Calories: 200
- Protein: 12g
- Carbohydrates: 3g
- Dietary Fiber: 1g
- Sugars: 1g
- Fat: 16g
- Saturated Fat: 3.5g
- Sodium: 160mg

Serves: 2

Cooking Time: 10 minutes

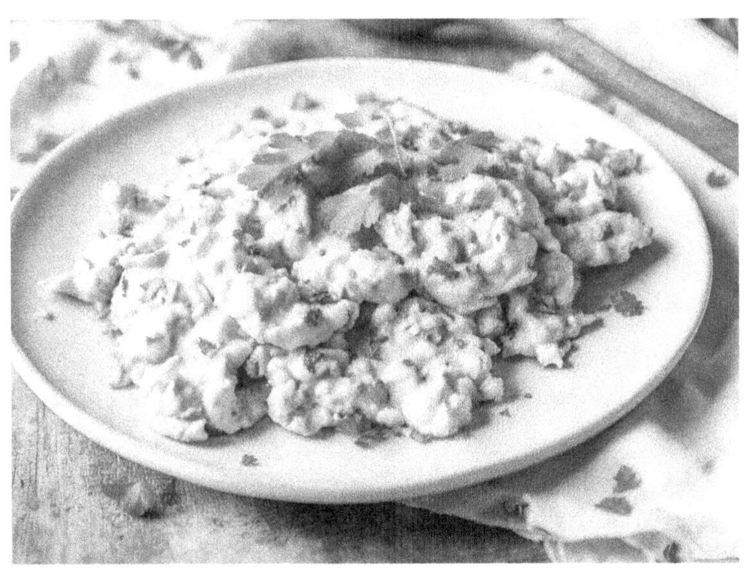

6. Sweet Potato Hash

Ingredients:

- 1 large sweet potato, peeled and diced
- 1/2 red bell pepper, diced
- 1/2 green bell pepper, diced
- 1/2 small red onion, diced
- 2 tablespoons olive oil
- 1 teaspoon smoked paprika
- 1/4 teaspoon garlic powder
- 1/4 teaspoon black pepper

Instructions:

1. Preheat the oven to 400°F (200°C).
2. In a large bowl, toss the diced sweet potato, bell peppers, and red onion with olive oil, smoked paprika, garlic powder, and black pepper.
3. Spread the mixture evenly on a baking sheet.
4. Roast for 25-30 minutes, stirring halfway through, until the sweet potatoes are tender and slightly crispy.
5. Serve immediately.

Nutrition Info (per serving):

- Calories: 180
- Protein: 2g
- Carbohydrates: 27g
- Dietary Fiber: 5g
- Sugars: 8g
- Fat: 7g
- Saturated Fat: 1g
- Sodium: 60mg

Serves: 2

Cooking Time: 35 minutes

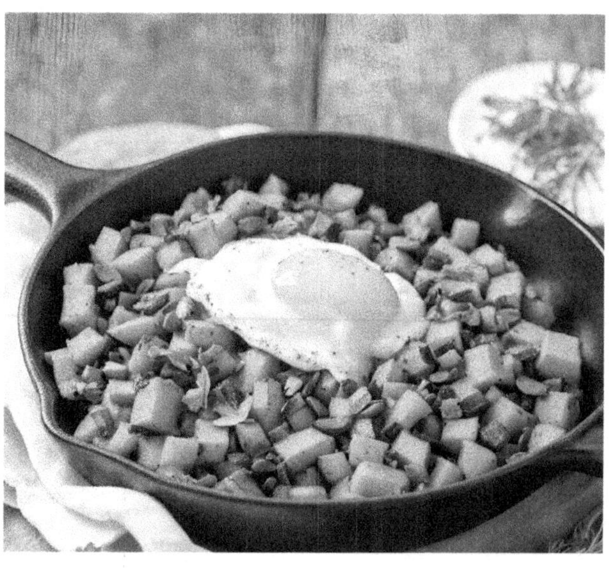

7. Buckwheat Pancakes

Ingredients:

- 1 cup buckwheat flour
- 1 tablespoon baking powder
- 1 tablespoon honey
- 1 cup unsweetened almond milk
- 1 large egg
- 1 teaspoon vanilla extract
- 2 tablespoons coconut oil, melted

Instructions:

1. In a large bowl, whisk together buckwheat flour and baking powder.
2. In another bowl, mix honey, almond milk, egg, vanilla extract, and melted coconut oil.
3. Pour the wet ingredients into the dry ingredients and stir until just combined.
4. Heat a non-stick skillet over medium heat and lightly grease with coconut oil.
5. Pour 1/4 cup of batter onto the skillet for each pancake. Cook until bubbles form on the surface, then flip and cook for another 1-2 minutes until golden brown.
6. Serve warm with your choice of toppings (fresh berries, maple syrup, etc.).

Nutrition Info (per serving):

- Calories: 250
- Protein: 6g
- Carbohydrates: 34g
- Dietary Fiber: 4g
- Sugars: 8g
- Fat: 10g
- Saturated Fat: 6g
- Sodium: 250mg

Serves: 4

Cooking Time: 20 minutes

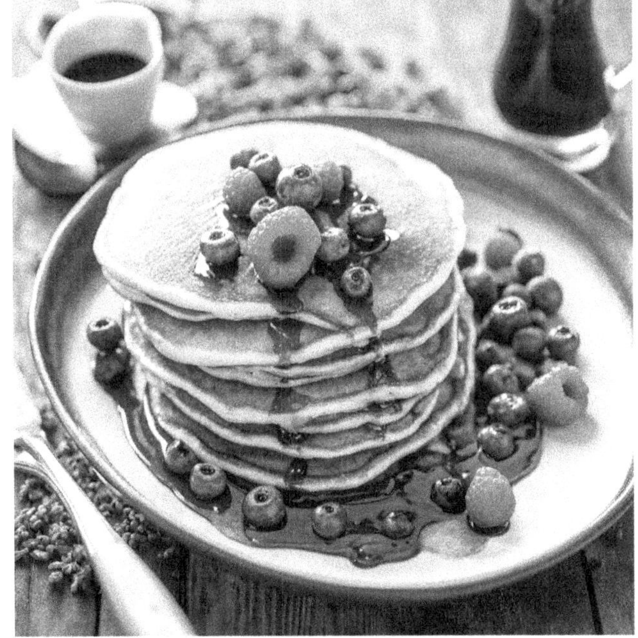

8. Spinach and Feta Omelet

Ingredients:

- 4 large eggs
- 1/4 cup unsweetened almond milk
- 1 tablespoon olive oil
- 1 cup fresh spinach leaves
- 1/4 cup crumbled feta cheese
- 1/4 teaspoon paprika

Instructions:

1. In a bowl, whisk together the eggs, almond milk, and paprika.
2. Heat olive oil in a non-stick skillet over medium heat.
3. Add the spinach and cook until wilted, about 2 minutes.
4. Pour the egg mixture into the skillet and cook until the edges start to set.
5. Sprinkle feta cheese over half of the omelet.
6. Fold the omelet in half and cook for another 2-3 minutes, until fully set.
7. Serve immediately.

Nutrition Info (per serving):

- Calories: 250
- Protein: 16g
- Carbohydrates: 3g
- Dietary Fiber: 1g
- Sugars: 1g
- Fat: 20g
- Saturated Fat: 6g
- Sodium: 380mg

Serves: 2

Cooking Time: 10 minutes

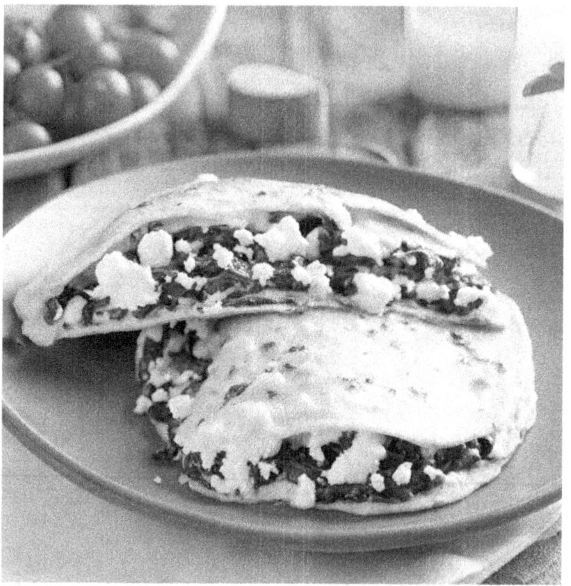

9. Mushroom and Herb Frittata

Ingredients:

- 8 large eggs
- 1/2 cup unsweetened almond milk
- 1 cup sliced mushrooms
- 1/4 cup chopped fresh herbs (parsley, chives, dill)
- 1 tablespoon olive oil
- 1/4 teaspoon garlic powder

Instructions:

1. Preheat the oven to 350°F (175°C).
2. In a bowl, whisk together the eggs, almond milk, and garlic powder.
3. Heat olive oil in an oven-safe skillet over medium heat.
4. Add the mushrooms and cook until softened, about 5 minutes.
5. Pour the egg mixture over the mushrooms and sprinkle with fresh herbs.
6. Transfer the skillet to the oven and bake for 15-20 minutes, until the frittata is set.
7. Slice and serve warm.

Nutrition Info (per serving):

- Calories: 180
- Protein: 14g
- Carbohydrates: 3g
- Dietary Fiber: 1g
- Sugars: 1g
- Fat: 12g
- Saturated Fat: 3g
- Sodium: 180mg

Serves: 4

Cooking Time: 30 minutes

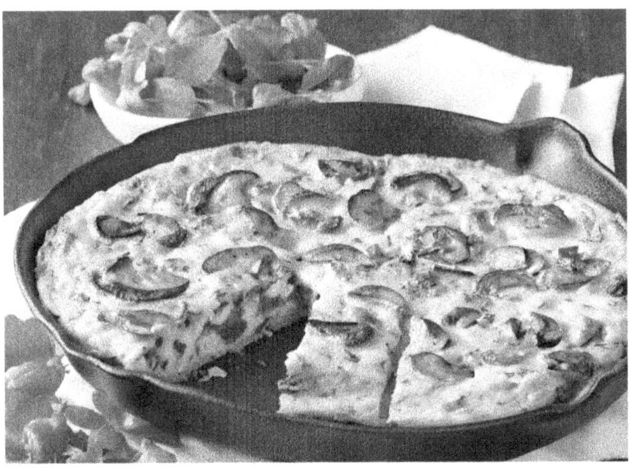

10. Zucchini and Bell Pepper Mini Quiches

Ingredients:

- 6 large eggs
- 1/2 cup unsweetened almond milk
- 1 cup grated zucchini
- 1/2 cup diced bell peppers (red, yellow, green)
- 1/4 cup shredded cheddar cheese
- 1 tablespoon olive oil
- 1/4 teaspoon dried oregano

Instructions:

1. Preheat the oven to 350°F (175°C) and grease a muffin tin with olive oil.
2. In a bowl, whisk together the eggs, almond milk, and oregano.
3. Stir in the grated zucchini, diced bell peppers, and cheddar cheese.
4. Pour the mixture evenly into the muffin tin cups.
5. Bake for 20-25 minutes, until the quiches are set and golden.
6. Allow to cool slightly before removing from the tin. Serve warm.

Nutrition Info (per serving):

- Calories: 120
- Protein: 8g
- Carbohydrates: 3g
- Dietary Fiber: 1g
- Sugars: 1g
- Fat: 9g
- Saturated Fat: 3g
- Sodium: 140mg

Serves: 6

Cooking Time: 30 minutes

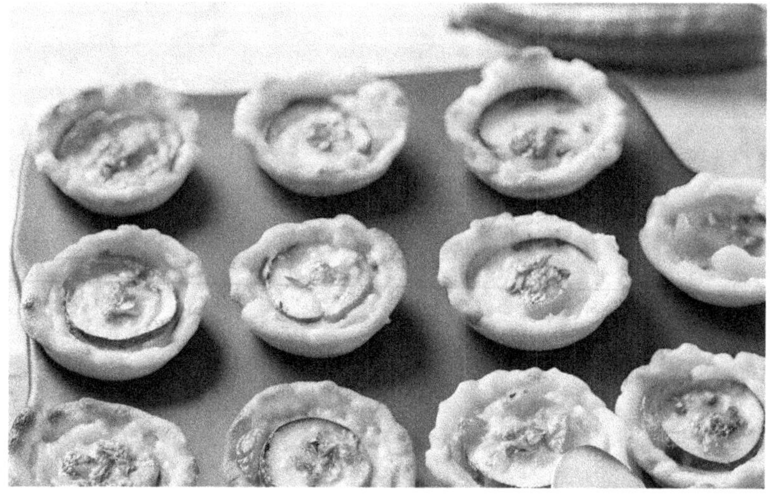

11. Avocado Egg Bake

Ingredients:

- 2 ripe avocados
- 4 large eggs
- 1/4 teaspoon paprika
- 1/4 teaspoon black pepper
- 1 tablespoon chopped chives

Instructions:

1. Preheat the oven to 425°F (220°C).
2. Cut the avocados in half and remove the pits.
3. Scoop out some of the flesh to create a larger well for the egg.
4. Place the avocado halves in a baking dish.
5. Crack an egg into each avocado half.
6. Sprinkle with paprika and black pepper.
7. Bake for 15-20 minutes, until the eggs are set.
8. Sprinkle with chopped chives before serving.

Nutrition Info (per serving):

- Calories: 220
- Protein: 9g
- Carbohydrates: 9g
- Dietary Fiber: 7g
- Sugars: 1g
- Fat: 18g
- Saturated Fat: 4g
- Sodium: 90mg

Serves: 2

Cooking Time: 20 minutes

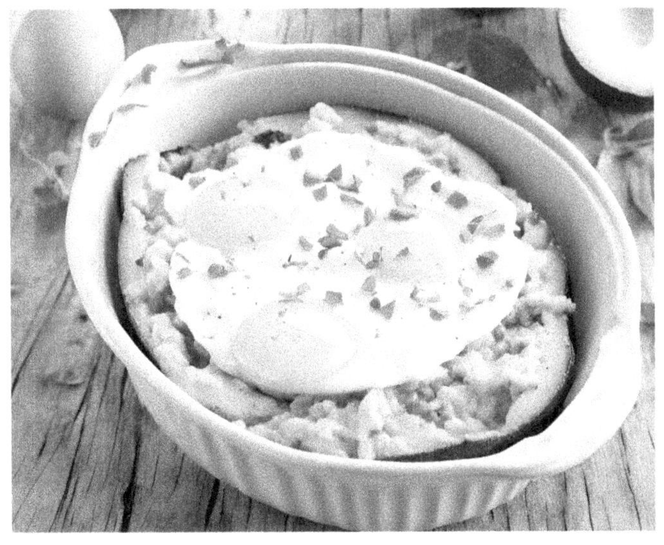

12. Tomato and Basil Egg Muffins

Ingredients:

- 6 large eggs
- 1/2 cup unsweetened almond milk
- 1/2 cup cherry tomatoes, halved
- 1/4 cup chopped fresh basil
- 1/4 cup grated Parmesan cheese
- 1 tablespoon olive oil
- 1/4 teaspoon garlic powder

Instructions:

1. Preheat the oven to 350°F (175°C) and grease a muffin tin with olive oil.
2. In a bowl, whisk together the eggs, almond milk, and garlic powder.
3. Stir in the cherry tomatoes, fresh basil, and Parmesan cheese.
4. Pour the mixture evenly into the muffin tin cups.
5. Bake for 20-25 minutes, until the muffins are set and golden.
6. Allow to cool slightly before removing from the tin. Serve warm.

Nutrition Info (per serving):

- Calories: 130
- Protein: 9g
- Carbohydrates: 3g
- Dietary Fiber: 1g
- Sugars: 1g
- Fat: 9g
- Saturated Fat: 3g
- Sodium: 150mg

Serves: 6

Cooking Time: 30 minutes

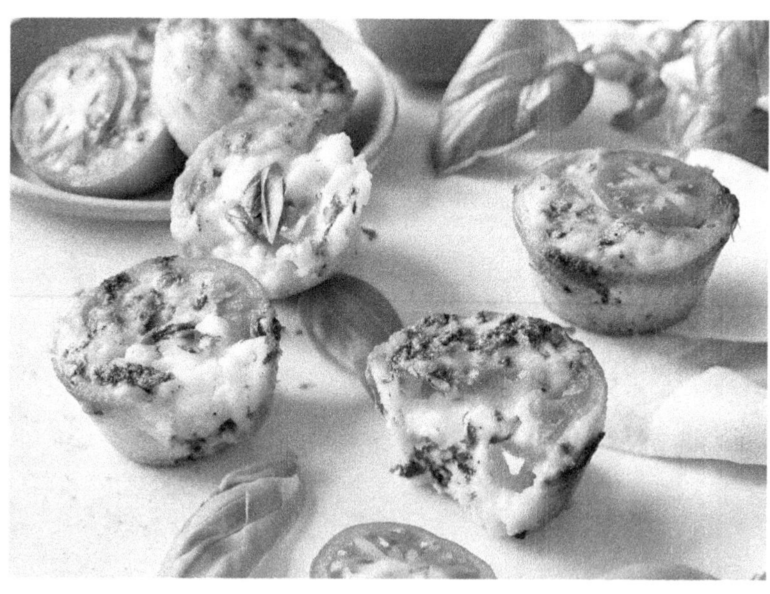

13. Berry Almond Breakfast Quinoa

Ingredients:

- 1 cup quinoa, rinsed
- 2 cups unsweetened almond milk
- 1 tablespoon honey
- 1 teaspoon vanilla extract
- 1/2 teaspoon ground cinnamon
- 1/2 cup fresh berries (blueberries, strawberries, raspberries)
- 1/4 cup sliced almonds

Instructions:

1. In a medium saucepan, combine quinoa and almond milk. Bring to a boil over medium heat.
2. Reduce heat to low and simmer, covered, for about 15 minutes or until the quinoa is tender and the liquid is absorbed.
3. Stir in the honey, vanilla extract, and cinnamon.
4. Divide into bowls and top with fresh berries and sliced almonds.

Nutrition Info (per serving):

- Calories: 280
- Protein: 8g
- Carbohydrates: 45g
- Dietary Fiber: 5g
- Sugars: 10g
- Fat: 8g
- Saturated Fat: 0.5g
- Sodium: 80mg

Serves: 2

Cooking Time: 20 minutes

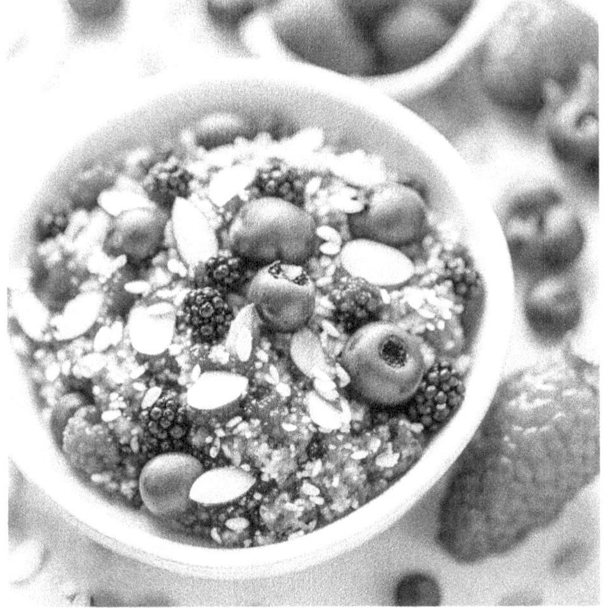

14. Overnight Oats with Pumpkin Seeds
Ingredients:

- 1 cup rolled oats
- 1 cup unsweetened almond milk
- 1/2 cup Greek yogurt
- 1 tablespoon honey
- 1/4 teaspoon cinnamon
- 1/4 cup pumpkin seeds
- 1/4 cup fresh berries

Instructions:

1. In a bowl, mix together rolled oats, almond milk, Greek yogurt, honey, and cinnamon.
2. Cover and refrigerate overnight.
3. In the morning, stir the oats and top with pumpkin seeds and fresh berries.
4. Serve chilled.

Nutrition Info (per serving):

- Calories: 250
- Protein: 10g
- Carbohydrates: 40g
- Dietary Fiber: 6g
- Sugars: 15g
- Fat: 8g
- Saturated Fat: 1g
- Sodium: 70mg

Serves: 2
Cooking Time: 5 minutes (plus overnight refrigeration)

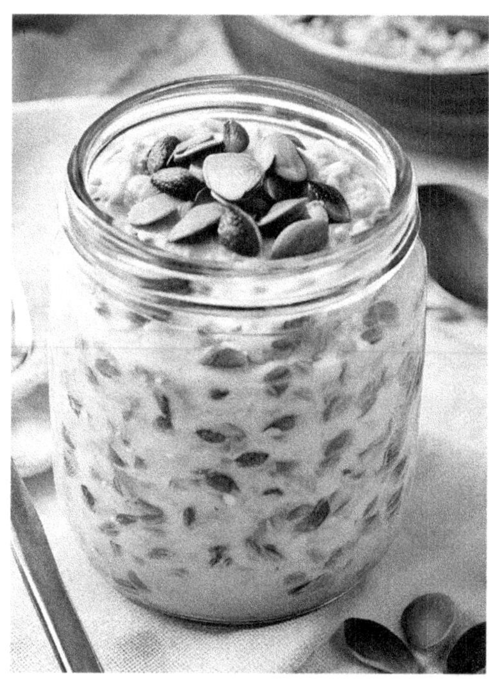

15. Smoked Salmon Breakfast Bowl

Ingredients:

- 1/2 cup cooked quinoa
- 1/4 cup diced cucumber
- 1/4 cup cherry tomatoes, halved
- 1/4 avocado, sliced
- 2 ounces smoked salmon
- 1 tablespoon olive oil
- 1 teaspoon lemon juice
- 1 tablespoon chopped dill

Instructions:

1. In a bowl, combine cooked quinoa, diced cucumber, cherry tomatoes, and avocado slices.
2. Top with smoked salmon.
3. Drizzle with olive oil and lemon juice.
4. Sprinkle with chopped dill before serving.

Nutrition Info (per serving):

- Calories: 320
- Protein: 15g
- Carbohydrates: 20g
- Dietary Fiber: 5g
- Sugars: 3g
- Fat: 20g
- Saturated Fat: 3g
- Sodium: 450mg

Serves: 1
Cooking Time: 10 minutes

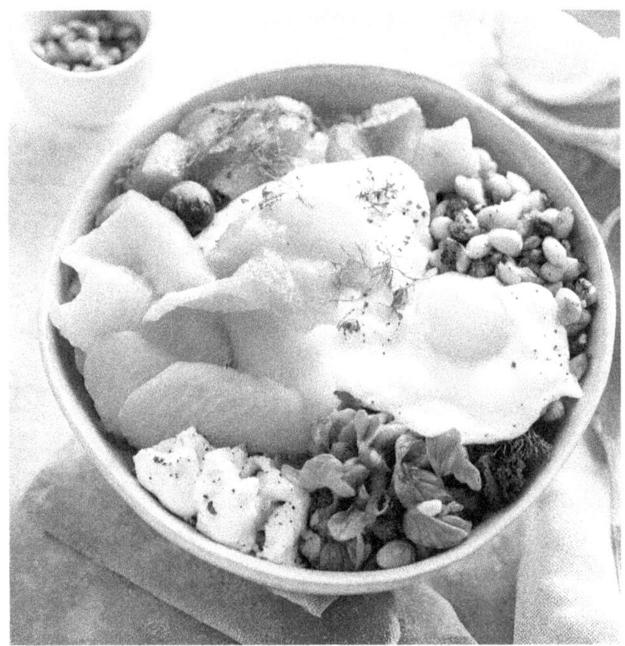

16. Almond Butter and Banana Toast

Ingredients:

- 2 slices whole grain bread
- 2 tablespoons almond butter
- 1 banana, sliced
- 1/4 teaspoon cinnamon

Instructions:

1. Toast the bread slices.
2. Spread almond butter evenly over the toasted bread.
3. Top with banana slices.
4. Sprinkle with cinnamon before serving.

Nutrition Info (per serving):

- Calories: 350
- Protein: 10g
- Carbohydrates: 45g
- Dietary Fiber: 7g
- Sugars: 15g
- Fat: 16g
- Saturated Fat: 1.5g
- Sodium: 180mg

Serves: 1

Cooking Time: 5 minutes

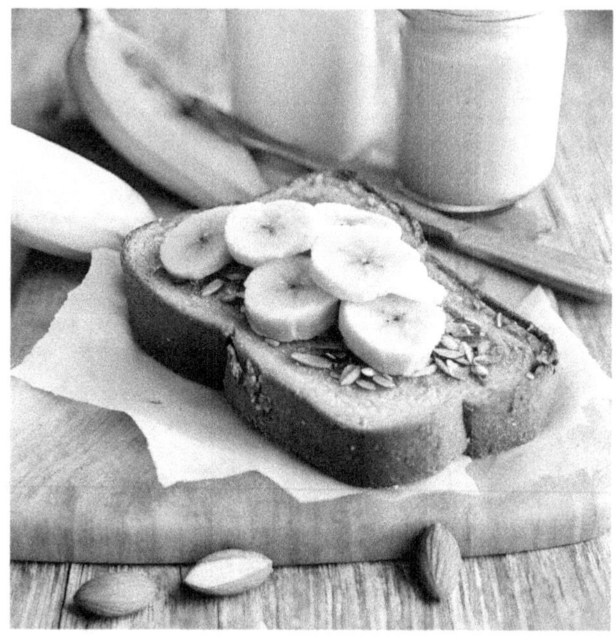

17. Nutty Rice Cakes

Ingredients:

- 2 rice cakes
- 2 tablespoons almond butter
- 1 tablespoon chopped walnuts
- 1 tablespoon chia seeds
- 1 teaspoon honey

Instructions:

1. Spread almond butter evenly over the rice cakes.
2. Sprinkle with chopped walnuts and chia seeds.
3. Drizzle with honey before serving.

Nutrition Info (per serving):

- Calories: 220
- Protein: 6g
- Carbohydrates: 25g
- Dietary Fiber: 4g
- Sugars: 8g
- Fat: 12g
- Saturated Fat: 1.5g
- Sodium: 50mg

Serves: 1

Cooking Time: 5 minutes

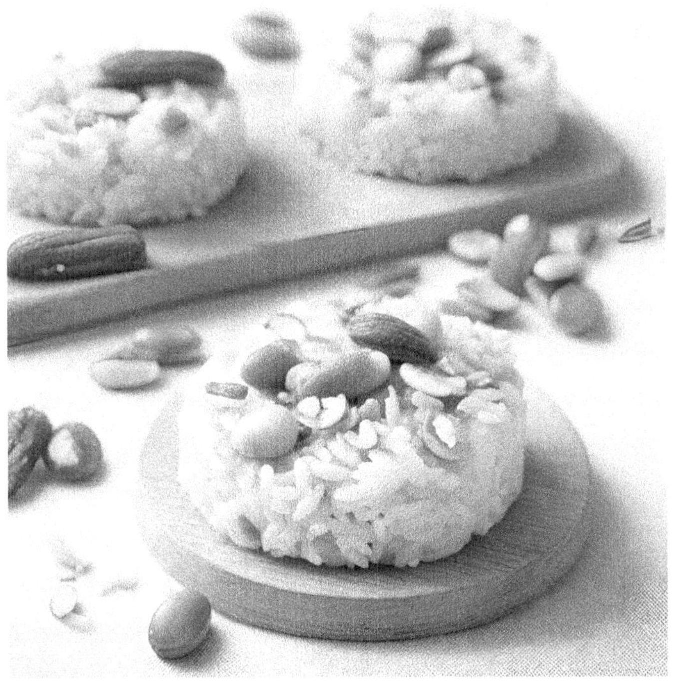

18. Baked Pear with Walnuts

Ingredients:

- 2 ripe pears, halved and cored
- 1/4 cup chopped walnuts
- 2 tablespoons honey
- 1/2 teaspoon ground cinnamon

Instructions:

1. Preheat the oven to 350°F (175°C).
2. Place the pear halves in a baking dish, cut side up.
3. Sprinkle with chopped walnuts and cinnamon.
4. Drizzle with honey.
5. Bake for 20-25 minutes, until the pears are tender.
6. Serve warm.

Nutrition Info (per serving):

- Calories: 180
- Protein: 2g
- Carbohydrates: 28g
- Dietary Fiber: 4g
- Sugars: 20g
- Fat: 8g
- Saturated Fat: 0.5g
- Sodium: 0mg

Serves: 2

Cooking Time: 30 minutes

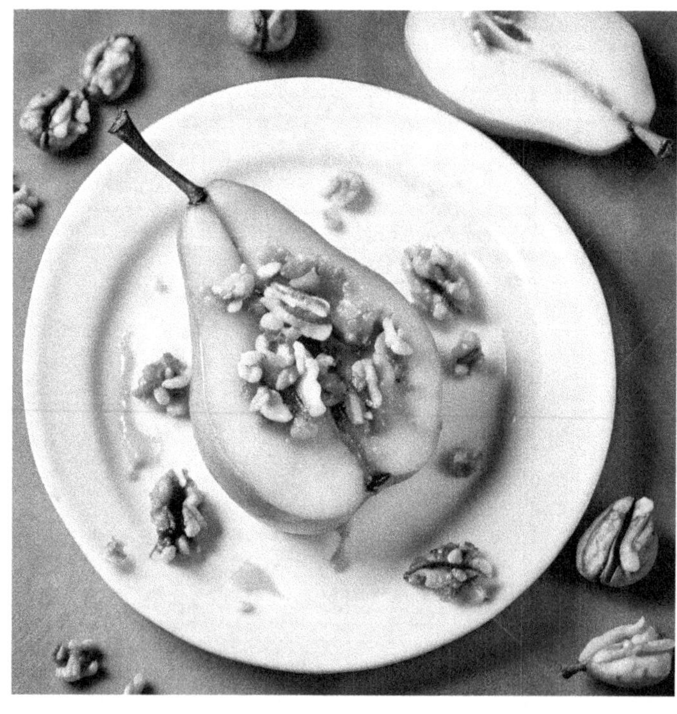

19. Savory Vegetable Muffins

Ingredients:

- 1 cup whole wheat flour
- 1/2 cup grated zucchini
- 1/2 cup grated carrot
- 1/4 cup chopped spinach
- 1/4 cup olive oil
- 2 large eggs
- 1/2 cup unsweetened almond milk
- 1 teaspoon baking powder
- 1/2 teaspoon dried thyme
- 1/2 teaspoon garlic powder

Instructions:

1. Preheat the oven to 375°F (190°C) and grease a muffin tin.
2. In a large bowl, whisk together the flour, baking powder, thyme, and garlic powder.
3. In another bowl, beat the eggs and mix in the olive oil and almond milk.
4. Combine the wet and dry ingredients, then fold in the grated zucchini, carrot, and spinach.
5. Pour the mixture into the muffin tin.
6. Bake for 20-25 minutes, until a toothpick inserted into the center comes out clean.
7. Allow to cool slightly before removing from the tin. Serve warm.

Nutrition Info (per serving):

- Calories: 150
- Protein: 4g
- Carbohydrates: 12g
- Dietary Fiber: 2g
- Sugars: 3g
- Fat: 10g
- Saturated Fat: 1.5g
- Sodium: 90mg

Serves: 12

Cooking Time: 30 minutes

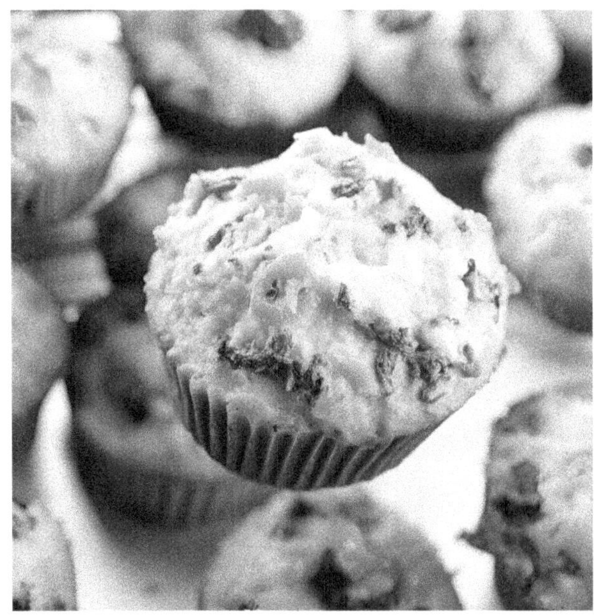

20. Polenta with Roasted Vegetables

Ingredients:

- 1 cup cornmeal
- 4 cups water
- 1 tablespoon olive oil
- 1 cup diced bell peppers (red, yellow, green)
- 1 cup cherry tomatoes, halved
- 1/2 cup diced zucchini
- 1/4 teaspoon paprika
- 1/4 teaspoon garlic powder

Instructions:

1. Preheat the oven to 400°F (200°C).
2. Toss the bell peppers, cherry tomatoes, and zucchini with olive oil, paprika, and garlic powder.
3. Spread the vegetables on a baking sheet and roast for 20 minutes, until tender.
4. In a medium saucepan, bring water to a boil.
5. Gradually whisk in the cornmeal, reduce heat, and cook, stirring frequently, until thick and creamy, about 15 minutes.
6. Serve the polenta topped with the roasted vegetables.

Nutrition Info (per serving):

- Calories: 180
- Protein: 4g
- Carbohydrates: 30g
- Dietary Fiber: 4g
- Sugars: 5g
- Fat: 5g
- Saturated Fat: 0.5g
- Sodium: 20mg

Serves: 4

Cooking Time: 35 minutes

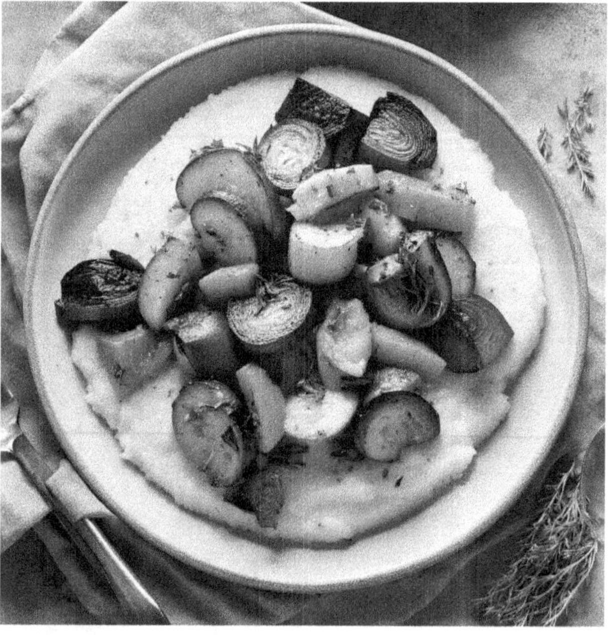

21. Matcha Green Tea Latte

Ingredients:

- 1 teaspoon matcha green tea powder
- 1 cup unsweetened almond milk
- 1 teaspoon honey
- 1/4 teaspoon vanilla extract

Instructions:

1. In a small bowl, whisk the matcha powder with a few tablespoons of hot water until smooth.
2. Heat the almond milk in a small saucepan over medium heat until hot but not boiling.
3. Remove from heat and whisk in the honey and vanilla extract.
4. Pour the almond milk into a cup and stir in the matcha mixture.
5. Serve warm.

Nutrition Info (per serving):

- Calories: 70
- Protein: 1g
- Carbohydrates: 10g
- Dietary Fiber: 1g
- Sugars: 8g
- Fat: 3g
- Saturated Fat: 0.5g
- Sodium: 80mg

Serves: 1

Cooking Time: 5 minutes

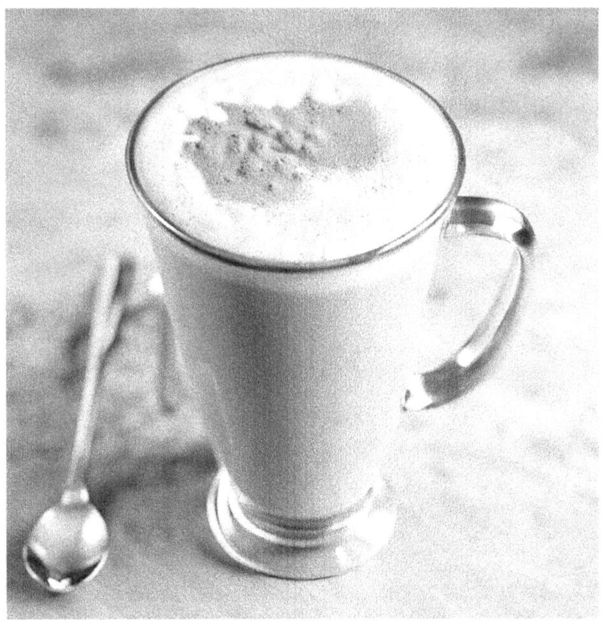

Fish Recipes

1. Mackerel Pâté

Ingredients:

- 200g smoked mackerel fillets, skin removed
- 100g cream cheese
- 2 tablespoons Greek yogurt
- 1 tablespoon lemon juice
- 1 tablespoon chopped fresh dill
- 1/2 teaspoon smoked paprika

Instructions:

1. Flake the mackerel fillets into a food processor.
2. Add cream cheese, Greek yogurt, lemon juice, dill, and smoked paprika.
3. Blend until smooth and creamy.
4. Transfer to a serving dish and refrigerate for at least 1 hour before serving.

Nutrition Info (per serving):

- Calories: 200
- Protein: 15g
- Carbohydrates: 3g
- Dietary Fiber: 0g
- Sugars: 2g
- Fat: 14g
- Saturated Fat: 6g
- Sodium: 300mg

Serves: 4

Cooking Time: 10 minutes (plus 1 hour refrigeration)

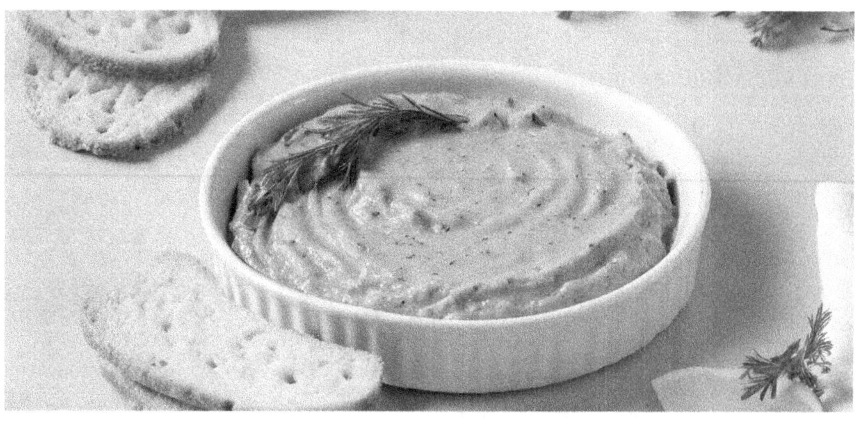

2. Smoked Trout Salad

Ingredients:

- 200g smoked trout fillets, flaked
- 4 cups mixed salad greens
- 1/2 cup cherry tomatoes, halved
- 1/2 cucumber, sliced
- 1/4 red onion, thinly sliced
- 2 tablespoons olive oil
- 1 tablespoon lemon juice
- 1 teaspoon Dijon mustard
- 1 tablespoon chopped fresh chives

Instructions:

1. In a small bowl, whisk together olive oil, lemon juice, and Dijon mustard.
2. In a large salad bowl, combine salad greens, cherry tomatoes, cucumber, and red onion.
3. Drizzle the dressing over the salad and toss to coat.
4. Top with flaked smoked trout and sprinkle with fresh chives.
5. Serve immediately.

Nutrition Info (per serving):

- Calories: 220
- Protein: 15g
- Carbohydrates: 6g
- Dietary Fiber: 2g
- Sugars: 3g
- Fat: 15g
- Saturated Fat: 2g
- Sodium: 320mg

Serves: 2

Cooking Time: 10 minutes

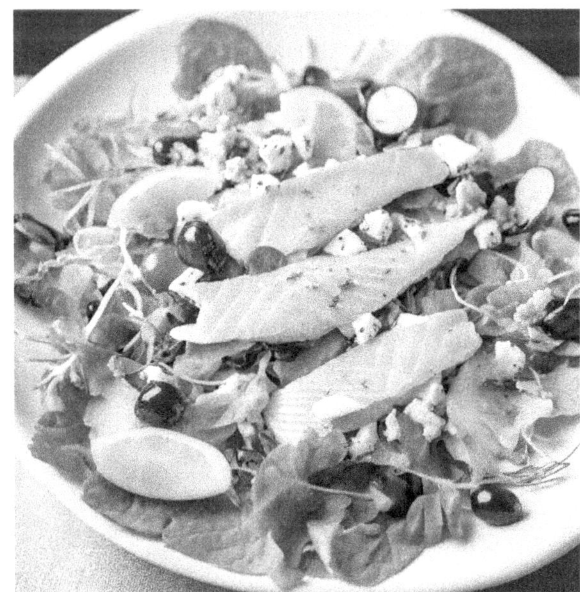

3. Ceviche with Tilapia

Ingredients:
- 400g fresh tilapia fillets, diced
- 1/2 cup fresh lime juice
- 1/2 cup fresh lemon juice
- 1/2 red onion, finely chopped
- 1 jalapeño, finely chopped
- 1/2 cup chopped cilantro
- 1 avocado, diced
- 1/2 cup diced tomatoes
- 1/4 teaspoon cumin

Instructions:
1. In a glass bowl, combine diced tilapia, lime juice, and lemon juice. Ensure the fish is fully submerged in the juice.
2. Cover and refrigerate for 2 hours, until the fish is opaque and "cooked" by the citrus juices.
3. Drain the fish and mix with red onion, jalapeño, cilantro, avocado, tomatoes, and cumin.
4. Serve chilled.

Nutrition Info (per serving):
- Calories: 180
- Protein: 22g
- Carbohydrates: 10g
- Dietary Fiber: 5g
- Sugars: 2g
- Fat: 6g
- Saturated Fat: 1g
- Sodium: 60mg

Serves: 4

Cooking Time: 2 hours (marinating time)

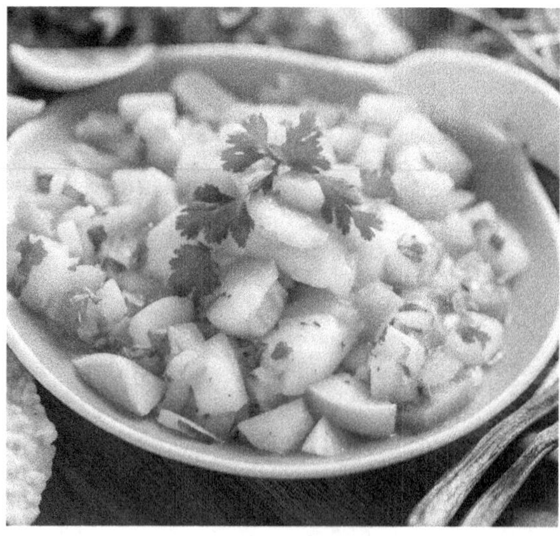

4. Salmon Nicoise Salad

Ingredients:

- 2 salmon fillets (about 200g each)
- 4 cups mixed salad greens
- 1/2 cup cherry tomatoes, halved
- 1/2 cup green beans, blanched
- 2 hard-boiled eggs, quartered
- 1/4 cup Kalamata olives
- 1/2 cup boiled baby potatoes, halved
- 2 tablespoons olive oil
- 1 tablespoon lemon juice
- 1 teaspoon Dijon mustard
- 1 tablespoon chopped fresh parsley

Instructions:

1. Preheat the oven to 375°F (190°C). Place salmon fillets on a baking sheet and bake for 15-20 minutes, until fully cooked.
2. In a small bowl, whisk together olive oil, lemon juice, and Dijon mustard.
3. In a large salad bowl, combine salad greens, cherry tomatoes, green beans, eggs, olives, and baby potatoes.
4. Drizzle with the dressing and toss gently.
5. Top with cooked salmon fillets and sprinkle with fresh parsley.
6. Serve immediately.

Nutrition Info (per serving):

- Calories: 350
- Protein: 28g
- Carbohydrates: 15g
- Dietary Fiber: 4g
- Sugars: 3g
- Fat: 20g
- Saturated Fat: 4g
- Sodium: 320mg

Serves: 2
Cooking Time: 25 minutes

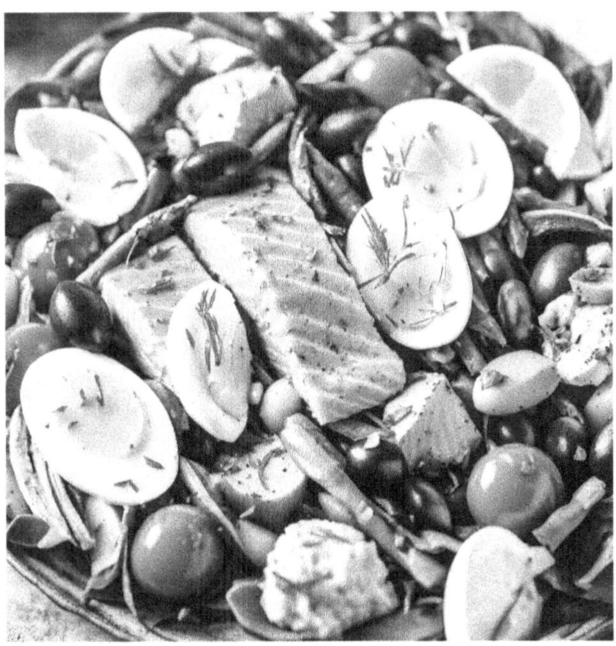

5. Thai Coconut Fish Soup

Ingredients:

- 400g white fish fillets (such as cod or tilapia), cut into chunks
- 1 can (400ml) coconut milk
- 2 cups fish or vegetable broth
- 1 tablespoon red curry paste
- 1 tablespoon fish sauce
- 1 tablespoon lime juice
- 1 red bell pepper, thinly sliced
- 1 cup sliced mushrooms
- 1 cup spinach leaves
- 2 tablespoons chopped fresh cilantro

Instructions:

1. In a large pot, bring coconut milk and broth to a simmer over medium heat.
2. Stir in red curry paste, fish sauce, and lime juice.
3. Add the red bell pepper and mushrooms, simmering for 5 minutes.
4. Add the fish chunks and simmer for another 5 minutes, until the fish is cooked through.
5. Stir in spinach leaves and cook until wilted, about 1 minute.
6. Garnish with fresh cilantro and serve hot.

Nutrition Info (per serving):

- Calories: 280
- Protein: 25g
- Carbohydrates: 10g
- Dietary Fiber: 3g
- Sugars: 3g
- Fat: 16g
- Saturated Fat: 12g
- Sodium: 700mg

Serves: 4

Cooking Time: 20 minutes

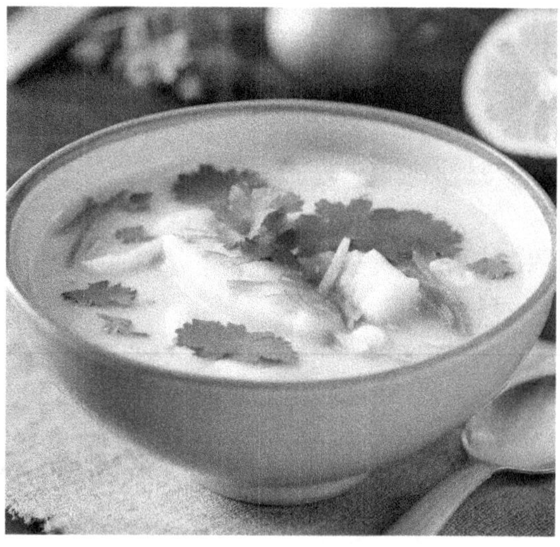

6. Mediterranean Fish Stew

Ingredients:

- 400g white fish fillets (such as cod or halibut), cut into chunks
- 2 tablespoons olive oil
- 1 onion, chopped
- 2 cloves garlic, minced
- 1 can (400g) diced tomatoes
- 1 cup fish or vegetable broth
- 1/2 cup sliced black olives
- 1/2 cup chopped fresh parsley
- 1 teaspoon dried oregano
- 1/4 teaspoon red pepper flakes

Instructions:

1. Heat olive oil in a large pot over medium heat. Add onion and garlic, cooking until softened, about 5 minutes.
2. Stir in diced tomatoes, broth, olives, parsley, oregano, and red pepper flakes.
3. Bring to a simmer and cook for 10 minutes.
4. Add the fish chunks and simmer for another 10 minutes, until the fish is cooked through.
5. Serve hot, garnished with additional parsley if desired.

Nutrition Info (per serving):

- Calories: 250
- Protein: 22g
- Carbohydrates: 10g
- Dietary Fiber: 2g
- Sugars: 5g
- Fat: 12g
- Saturated Fat: 2g
- Sodium: 600mg

Serves: 4

Cooking Time: 30 minutes

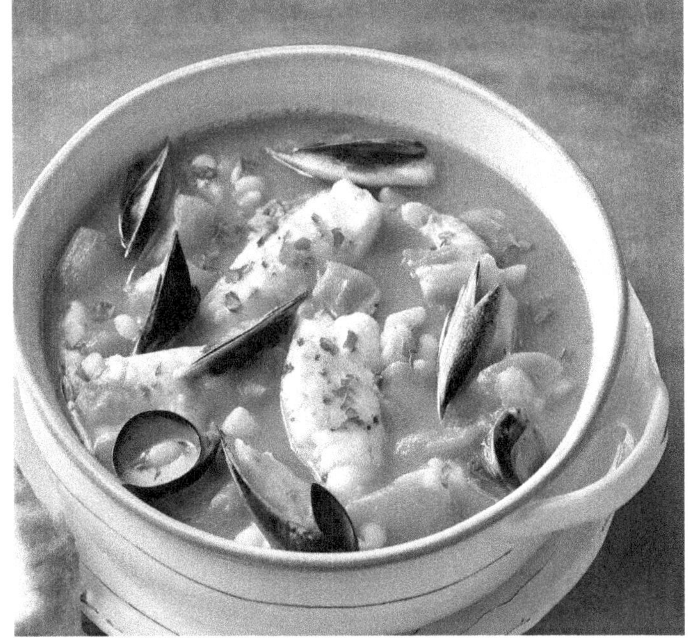

7. Salmon Chowder

Ingredients:

- 400g salmon fillets, skinned and diced
- 2 tablespoons olive oil
- 1 onion, chopped
- 2 cloves garlic, minced
- 2 cups fish or vegetable broth
- 1 cup unsweetened almond milk
- 2 potatoes, peeled and diced
- 1 cup corn kernels (fresh or frozen)
- 1 teaspoon dried thyme
- 1 tablespoon lemon juice

Instructions:

1. Heat olive oil in a large pot over medium heat. Add onion and garlic, cooking until softened, about 5 minutes.
2. Add the broth, almond milk, and potatoes. Bring to a simmer and cook for 10 minutes.
3. Stir in the corn, thyme, and lemon juice. Simmer for another 5 minutes.
4. Add the salmon and cook for an additional 5 minutes, until the salmon is cooked through.
5. Serve hot.

Nutrition Info (per serving):

- Calories: 320
- Protein: 25g
- Carbohydrates: 20g
- Dietary Fiber: 3g
- Sugars: 4g
- Fat: 16g
- Saturated Fat: 2.5g
- Sodium: 350mg

Serves: 4

Cooking Time: 30 minutes

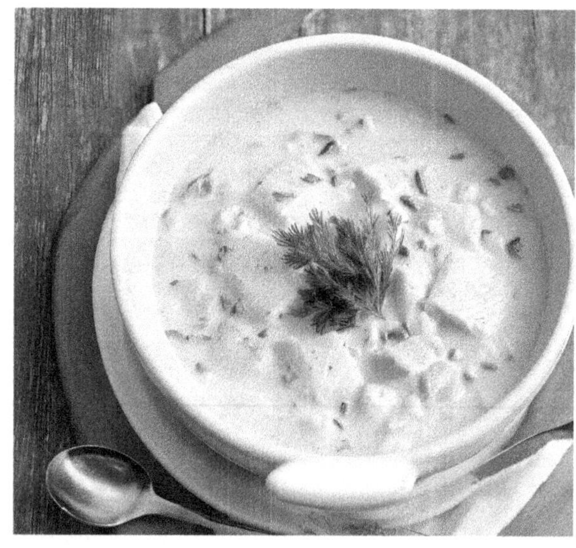

8. Saffron Poached Haddock

Ingredients:

- 400g haddock fillets
- 2 cups fish or vegetable broth
- 1/2 cup dry white wine
- 1/2 onion, thinly sliced
- 1 clove garlic, minced
- 1 teaspoon saffron threads
- 1 tablespoon lemon juice
- 1 tablespoon chopped fresh parsley

Instructions:

1. In a large skillet, combine broth, wine, onion, garlic, and saffron. Bring to a simmer over medium heat.
2. Add the haddock fillets and poach for 8-10 minutes, until the fish is opaque and flakes easily with a fork.
3. Remove the fish and place on a serving dish.
4. Stir lemon juice into the poaching liquid and reduce for 2-3 minutes.
5. Pour the sauce over the haddock and garnish with chopped parsley.
6. Serve immediately.

Nutrition Info (per serving):

- Calories: 200
- Protein: 28g
- Carbohydrates: 3g
- Dietary Fiber: 1g
- Sugars: 1g
- Fat: 6g
- Saturated Fat: 1g
- Sodium: 320mg

Serves: 4

Cooking Time: 20 minutes

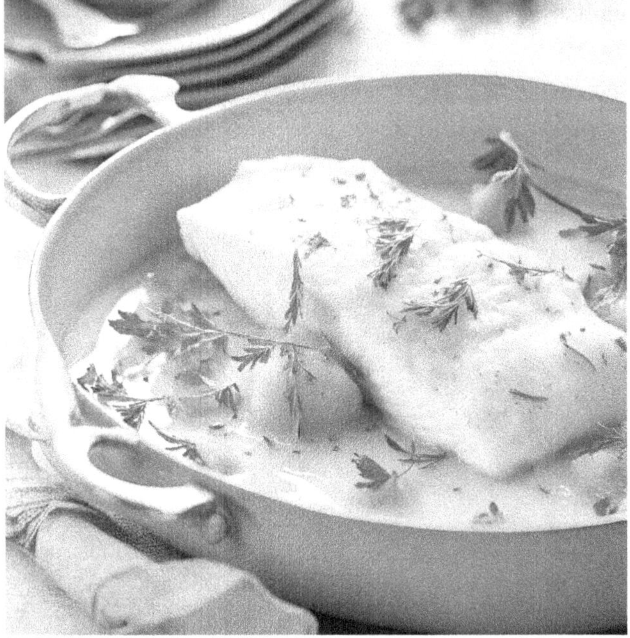

9. Miso Poached Tilapia

Ingredients:

- 4 tilapia fillets
- 4 cups water
- 1/4 cup white miso paste
- 1 tablespoon soy sauce
- 1-inch piece ginger, sliced
- 2 green onions, chopped
- 1 cup baby spinach

Instructions:

1. In a large saucepan, bring water, miso paste, soy sauce, and ginger to a simmer.
2. Add the tilapia fillets and poach for 8-10 minutes until the fish is opaque and flakes easily.
3. Remove the fish and set aside.
4. Add the spinach to the broth and cook until wilted, about 1 minute.
5. Serve the tilapia fillets over the wilted spinach, garnished with green onions.

Nutrition Info (per serving):

- Calories: 180
- Protein: 30g
- Carbohydrates: 4g
- Dietary Fiber: 1g
- Sugars: 1g
- Fat: 3g
- Saturated Fat: 0.5g
- Sodium: 600mg

Serves: 4

Cooking Time: 15 minutes

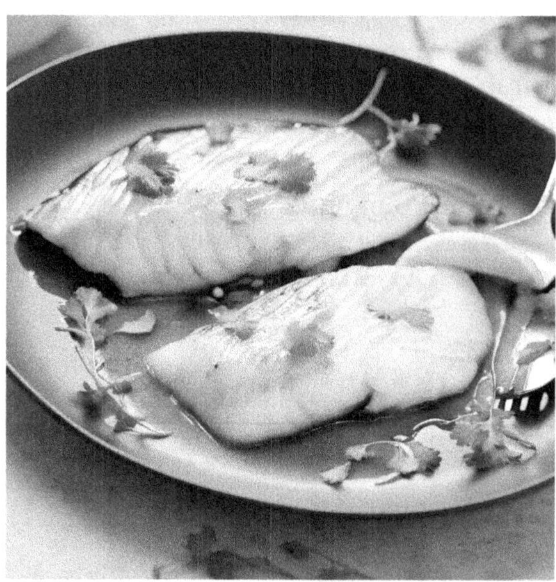

10. Herbal Steamed Snapper

Ingredients:

- 4 snapper fillets
- 1 lemon, thinly sliced
- 2 sprigs fresh rosemary
- 2 sprigs fresh thyme
- 1/4 cup white wine
- 1/2 cup vegetable broth
- 1 tablespoon olive oil

Instructions:

1. Place a steaming basket over a pot with white wine and vegetable broth. Bring to a simmer.
2. Arrange lemon slices, rosemary, and thyme on the snapper fillets.
3. Place the fillets in the steaming basket and cover.
4. Steam for 8-10 minutes until the fish is opaque and flakes easily.
5. Drizzle with olive oil before serving.

Nutrition Info (per serving):

- Calories: 200
- Protein: 30g
- Carbohydrates: 3g
- Dietary Fiber: 1g
- Sugars: 1g
- Fat: 6g
- Saturated Fat: 1g
- Sodium: 150mg

Serves: 4

Cooking Time: 15 minutes

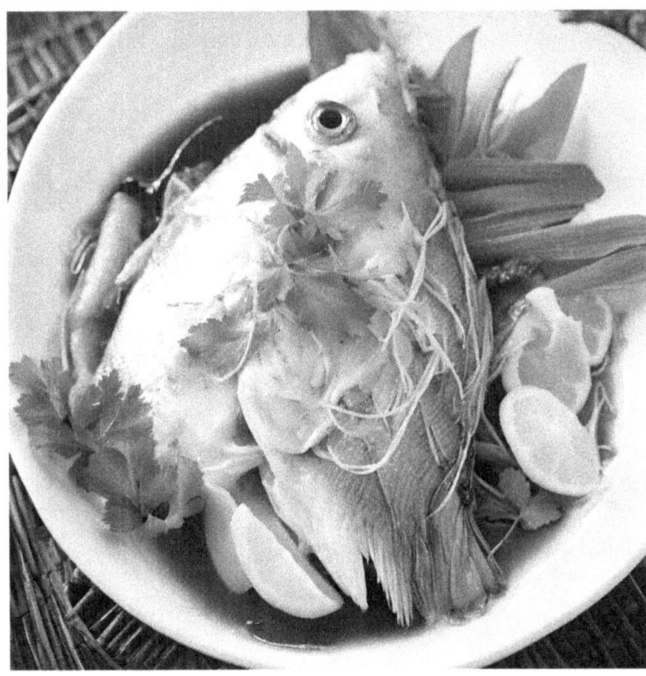

11. Fennel and Orange Steamed Trout
Ingredients:
- 4 trout fillets
- 1 bulb fennel, thinly sliced
- 1 orange, thinly sliced
- 1 tablespoon olive oil
- 1/4 teaspoon cumin
- 1/4 teaspoon coriander

Instructions:
1. Place a steaming basket over a pot with water. Bring to a simmer.
2. Arrange fennel and orange slices on the trout fillets.
3. Sprinkle with cumin and coriander.
4. Place the fillets in the steaming basket and cover.
5. Steam for 10-12 minutes until the fish is opaque and flakes easily.
6. Drizzle with olive oil before serving.

Nutrition Info (per serving):
- Calories: 210
- Protein: 28g
- Carbohydrates: 6g
- Dietary Fiber: 2g
- Sugars: 3g
- Fat: 8g
- Saturated Fat: 1.5g
- Sodium: 80mg

Serves: 4
Cooking Time: 20 minutes

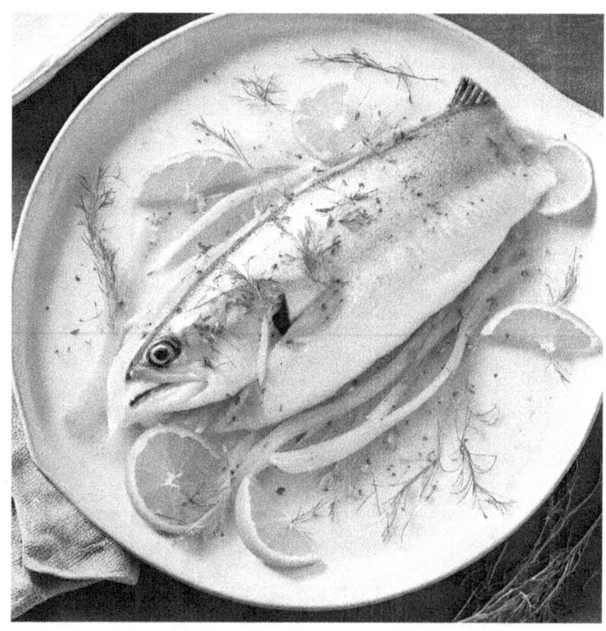

12. Lemon Thyme Poached Cod

Ingredients:

- 4 cod fillets
- 4 cups vegetable broth
- 1 lemon, sliced
- 4 sprigs fresh thyme
- 1 tablespoon olive oil

Instructions:

1. In a large saucepan, bring vegetable broth, lemon slices, and thyme to a simmer.
2. Add the cod fillets and poach for 8-10 minutes until the fish is opaque and flakes easily.
3. Remove the fish and set aside.
4. Drizzle with olive oil before serving.

Nutrition Info (per serving):

- Calories: 180
- Protein: 32g
- Carbohydrates: 3g
- Dietary Fiber: 1g
- Sugars: 1g
- Fat: 4g
- Saturated Fat: 0.5g
- Sodium: 300mg

Serves: 4

Cooking Time: 15 minutes

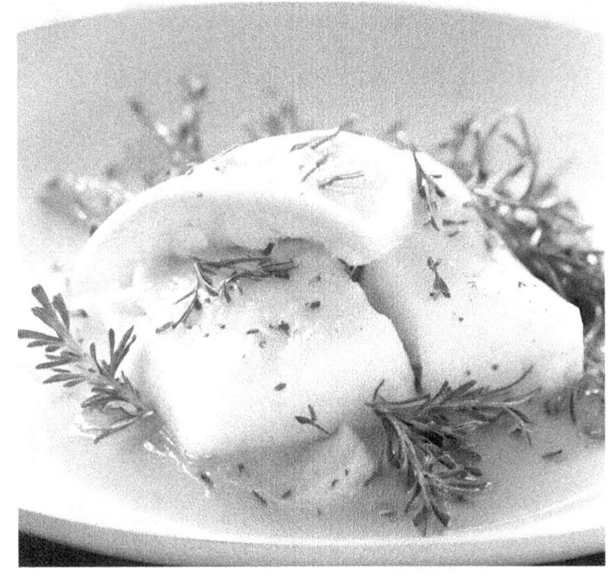

13. Steamed Halibut with Greens

Ingredients:

- 4 halibut fillets
- 1 cup vegetable broth
- 1/2 cup white wine
- 2 cups kale, chopped
- 1/4 cup lemon juice
- 1 tablespoon olive oil

Instructions:

1. Place a steaming basket over a pot with vegetable broth and white wine. Bring to a simmer.
2. Arrange the halibut fillets in the steaming basket and cover.
3. Steam for 10-12 minutes until the fish is opaque and flakes easily.
4. Meanwhile, sauté kale in olive oil until wilted, about 5 minutes.
5. Drizzle the fish with lemon juice before serving over the wilted kale.

Nutrition Info (per serving):

- Calories: 240
- Protein: 34g
- Carbohydrates: 5g
- Dietary Fiber: 2g
- Sugars: 1g
- Fat: 8g
- Saturated Fat: 1.5g
- Sodium: 350mg

Serves: 4

Cooking Time: 20 minutes

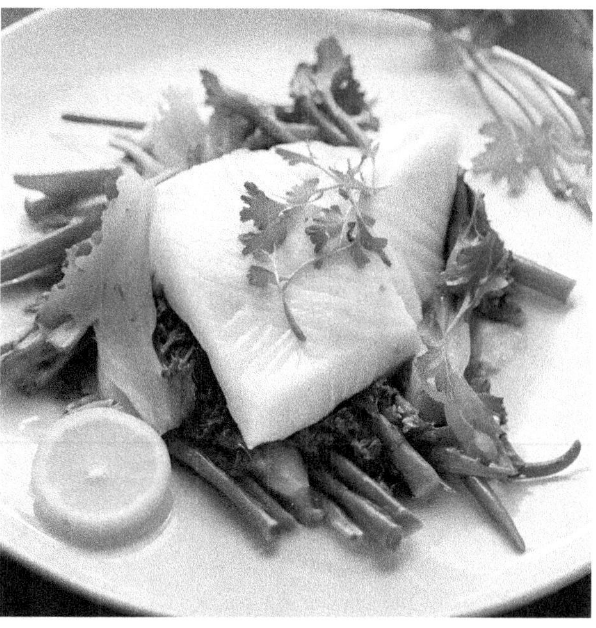

14. Ginger Soy Poached Salmon

Ingredients:

- 4 salmon fillets
- 4 cups vegetable broth
- 1/4 cup soy sauce
- 1-inch piece ginger, sliced
- 2 green onions, chopped
- 1 tablespoon sesame oil

Instructions:

1. In a large saucepan, bring vegetable broth, soy sauce, and ginger to a simmer.
2. Add the salmon fillets and poach for 10-12 minutes until the fish is opaque and flakes easily.
3. Remove the fish and set aside.
4. Drizzle with sesame oil and garnish with green onions before serving.

Nutrition Info (per serving):

- Calories: 300
- Protein: 28g
- Carbohydrates: 4g
- Dietary Fiber: 1g
- Sugars: 1g
- Fat: 20g
- Saturated Fat: 3.5g
- Sodium: 800mg

Serves: 4

Cooking Time: 15 minutes

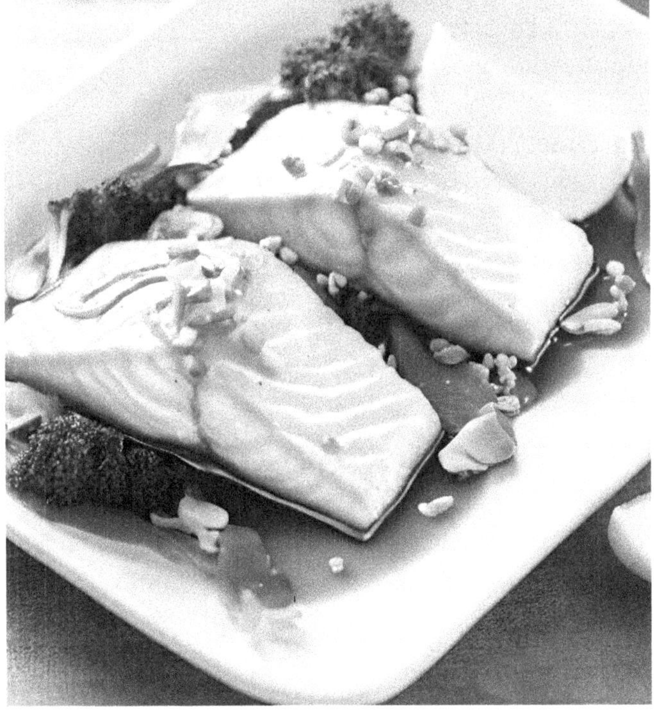

15. Spiced Catfish
Ingredients:
- 4 catfish fillets
- 1 tablespoon olive oil
- 1 teaspoon paprika
- 1/2 teaspoon cumin
- 1/2 teaspoon garlic powder

Instructions:
1. Preheat the oven to 400°F (200°C).
2. Brush the catfish fillets with olive oil.
3. In a small bowl, mix together paprika, cumin, and garlic powder.
4. Sprinkle the spice mixture evenly over both sides of the fish.
5. Place the fillets on a baking sheet and bake for 12-15 minutes until the fish is opaque and flakes easily.
6. Serve immediately.

Nutrition Info (per serving):
- Calories: 200
- Protein: 25g
- Carbohydrates: 2g
- Dietary Fiber: 1g
- Sugars: 0g
- Fat: 10g
- Saturated Fat: 2g
- Sodium: 100mg

Serves: 4
Cooking Time: 20 minutes

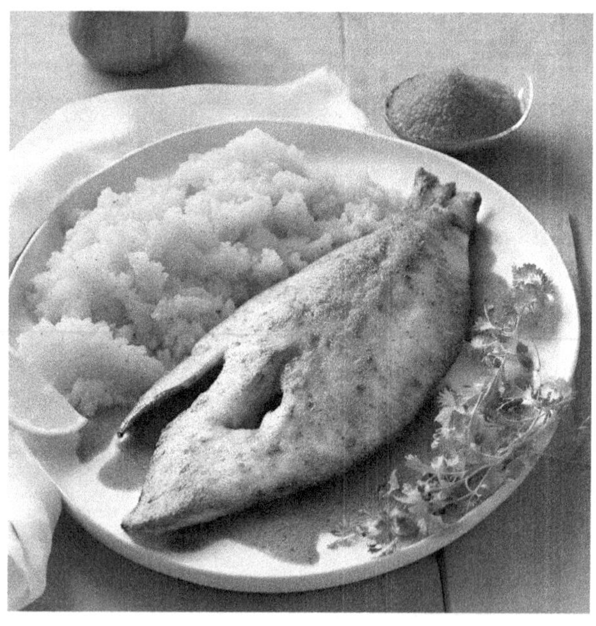

16. Caper and Dill Salmon Stir-Fry

Ingredients:

- 4 salmon fillets, cut into bite-sized pieces
- 2 tablespoons olive oil
- 1 cup cherry tomatoes, halved
- 1/4 cup capers, drained
- 1/4 cup chopped fresh dill
- 1 lemon, juiced

Instructions:

1. Heat olive oil in a large skillet over medium-high heat.
2. Add the salmon pieces and cook for 3-4 minutes until browned on all sides.
3. Add cherry tomatoes and capers, cooking for another 2-3 minutes until the tomatoes soften.
4. Stir in fresh dill and lemon juice.
5. Serve hot.

Nutrition Info (per serving):

- Calories: 250
- Protein: 25g
- Carbohydrates: 4g
- Dietary Fiber: 1g
- Sugars: 2g
- Fat: 15g
- Saturated Fat: 2.5g
- Sodium: 400mg

Serves: 4

Cooking Time: 15 minutes

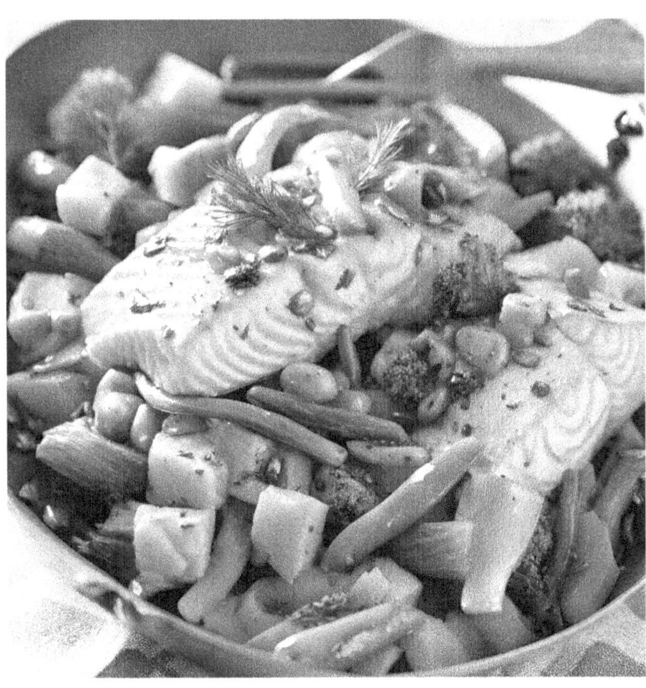

17. Mustard Crusted Trout

Ingredients:

- 4 trout fillets
- 2 tablespoons Dijon mustard
- 1/4 cup whole wheat breadcrumbs
- 1 tablespoon olive oil
- 1 teaspoon dried thyme

Instructions:

1. Preheat the oven to 375°F (190°C).
2. Brush the trout fillets with Dijon mustard.
3. In a small bowl, mix together breadcrumbs, olive oil, and dried thyme.
4. Press the breadcrumb mixture onto the top of each fillet.
5. Place the fillets on a baking sheet and bake for 12-15 minutes until the fish is opaque and flakes easily.
6. Serve immediately.

Nutrition Info (per serving):

- Calories: 220
- Protein: 24g
- Carbohydrates: 5g
- Dietary Fiber: 1g
- Sugars: 1g
- Fat: 12g
- Saturated Fat: 2.5g
- Sodium: 150mg

Serves: 4

Cooking Time: 20 minutes

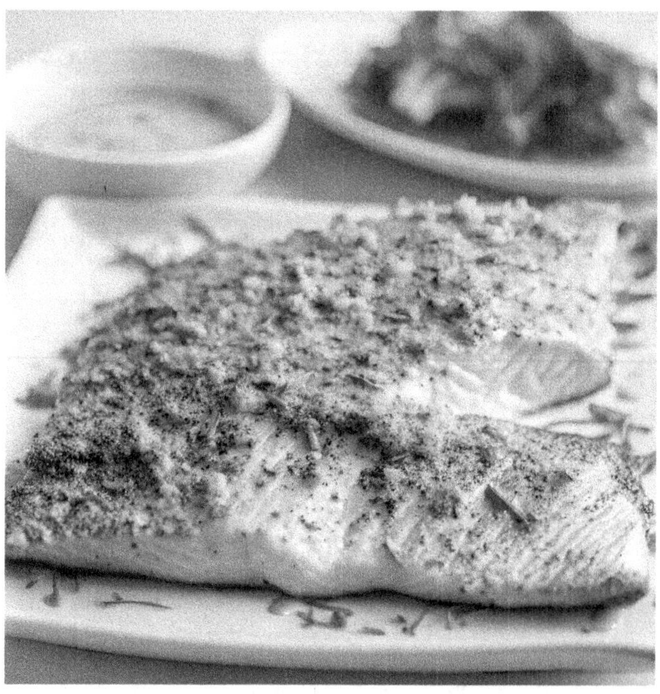

18. Chili Lime Cod

Ingredients:

- 4 cod fillets
- 2 tablespoons olive oil
- 1 lime, juiced
- 1 teaspoon chili powder
- 1/2 teaspoon garlic powder

Instructions:

1. Preheat the oven to 400°F (200°C).
2. In a small bowl, mix together olive oil, lime juice, chili powder, and garlic powder.
3. Brush the mixture onto both sides of the cod fillets.
4. Place the fillets on a baking sheet and bake for 12-15 minutes until the fish is opaque and flakes easily.
5. Serve immediately.

Nutrition Info (per serving):

- Calories: 180
- Protein: 30g
- Carbohydrates: 2g
- Dietary Fiber: 1g
- Sugars: 0g
- Fat: 5g
- Saturated Fat: 0.5g
- Sodium: 150mg

Serves: 4

Cooking Time: 20 minutes

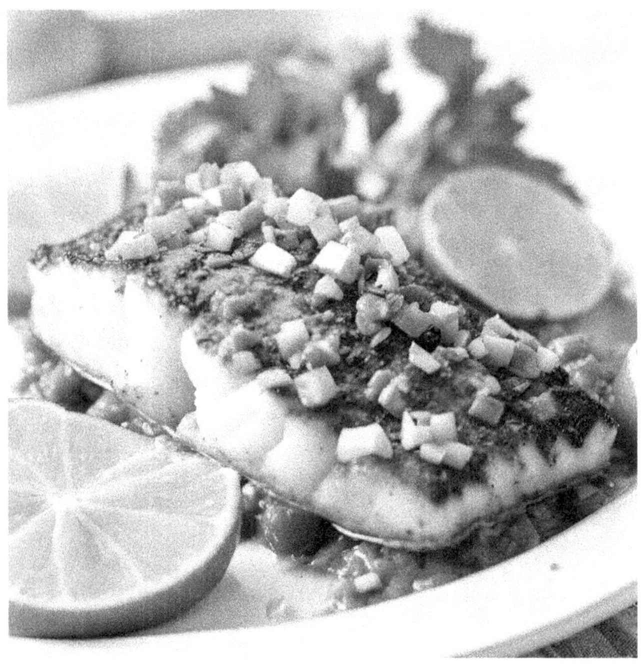

19. Lemon Pepper Flounder

Ingredients:

- 4 flounder fillets
- 1 tablespoon olive oil
- 1 lemon, zested and juiced
- 1 teaspoon black pepper

Instructions:

1. Preheat the oven to 375°F (190°C).
2. Brush the flounder fillets with olive oil.
3. In a small bowl, mix together lemon zest, lemon juice, and black pepper.
4. Brush the lemon mixture onto both sides of the fish.
5. Place the fillets on a baking sheet and bake for 10-12 minutes until the fish is opaque and flakes easily.
6. Serve immediately.

Nutrition Info (per serving):

- Calories: 160
- Protein: 28g
- Carbohydrates: 2g
- Dietary Fiber: 1g
- Sugars: 0g
- Fat: 4g
- Saturated Fat: 0.5g
- Sodium: 100mg

Serves: 4

Cooking Time: 15 minutes

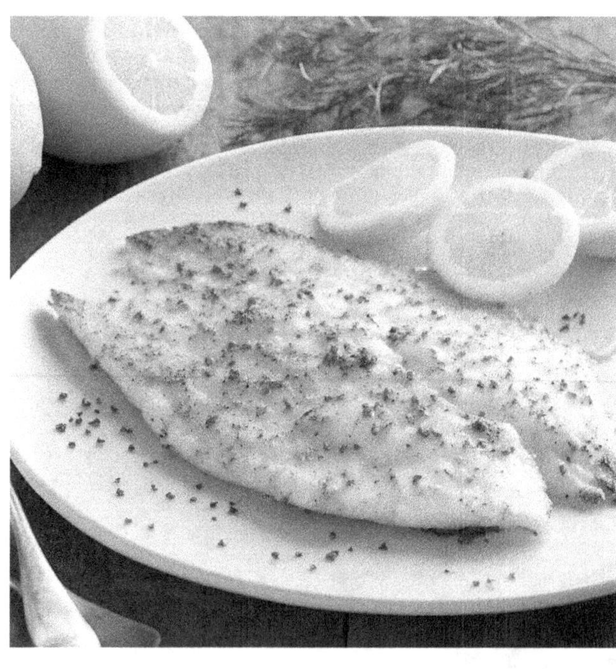

20. Sesame Crusted Tuna

Ingredients:

- 4 tuna steaks
- 1/4 cup sesame seeds
- 2 tablespoons soy sauce
- 1 tablespoon sesame oil
- 1 teaspoon grated ginger

Instructions:

1. In a small bowl, mix together soy sauce, sesame oil, and grated ginger.
2. Brush the mixture onto both sides of the tuna steaks.
3. Press sesame seeds onto both sides of the tuna steaks.
4. Heat a non-stick skillet over medium-high heat.
5. Cook the tuna steaks for 2-3 minutes per side for medium-rare.
6. Serve immediately.

Nutrition Info (per serving):

- Calories: 280
- Protein: 35g
- Carbohydrates: 3g
- Dietary Fiber: 1g
- Sugars: 0g
- Fat: 14g
- Saturated Fat: 2g
- Sodium: 500mg

Serves: 4

Cooking Time: 15 minutes

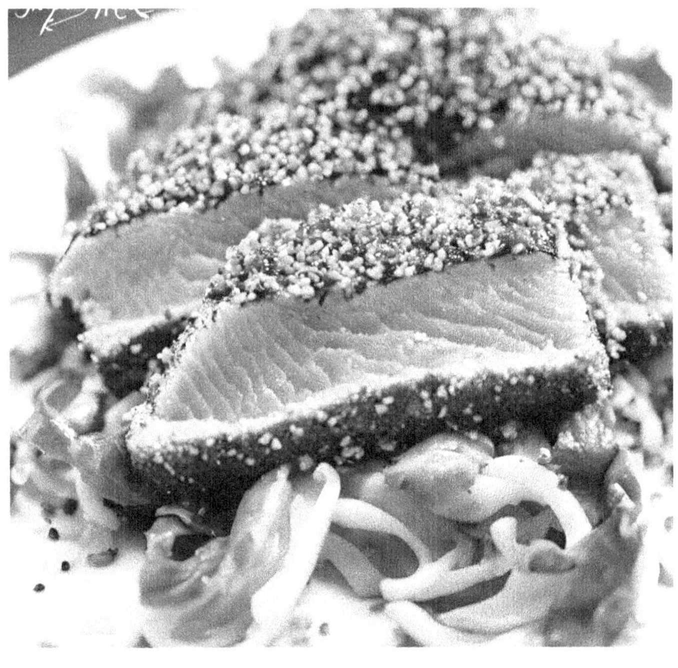

21. Garlic Lime Mahi Mahi

Ingredients:

- 4 mahi mahi fillets
- 2 tablespoons olive oil
- 2 cloves garlic, minced
- 1 lime, juiced
- 1/4 teaspoon paprika

Instructions:

1. Preheat the oven to 400°F (200°C).
2. In a small bowl, mix together olive oil, garlic, lime juice, and paprika.
3. Brush the mixture onto both sides of the mahi mahi fillets.
4. Place the fillets on a baking sheet and bake for 12-15 minutes until the fish is opaque and flakes easily.
5. Serve immediately.

Nutrition Info (per serving):

- Calories: 200
- Protein: 30g
- Carbohydrates: 2g
- Dietary Fiber: 1g
- Sugars: 0g
- Fat: 8g
- Saturated Fat: 1g
- Sodium: 150mg

Serves: 4

Cooking Time: 20 minutes

22. Mediterranean Baked Snapper

Ingredients:

- 4 snapper fillets
- 1/4 cup olive oil
- 1 lemon, sliced
- 1 cup cherry tomatoes, halved
- 1/4 cup Kalamata olives, halved
- 1 tablespoon chopped fresh parsley
- 1 teaspoon dried oregano

Instructions:

1. Preheat the oven to 375°F (190°C).
2. Place the snapper fillets in a baking dish.
3. Arrange lemon slices, cherry tomatoes, and olives around the fish.
4. Drizzle with olive oil and sprinkle with dried oregano.
5. Bake for 20-25 minutes until the fish is opaque and flakes easily.
6. Garnish with fresh parsley before serving.

Nutrition Info (per serving):

- Calories: 250
- Protein: 28g
- Carbohydrates: 5g
- Dietary Fiber: 1g
- Sugars: 2g
- Fat: 12g
- Saturated Fat: 2g
- Sodium: 300mg

Serves: 4

Cooking Time: 30 minutes

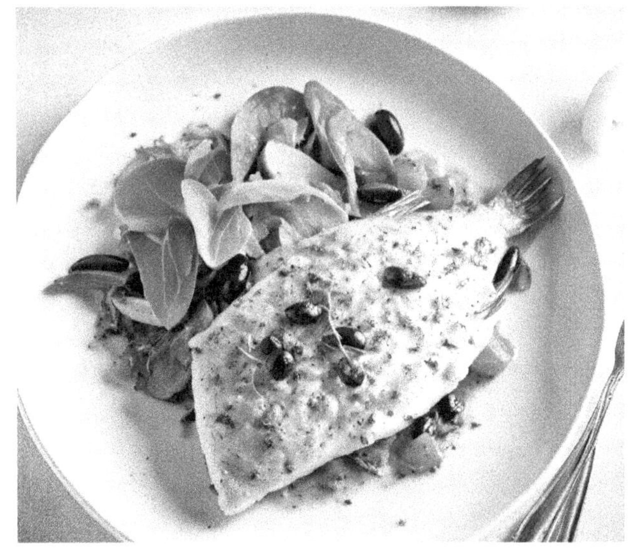

23. Grilled Sardines with Lemon and Herbs

Ingredients:

- 8 whole sardines, cleaned and gutted
- 1/4 cup olive oil
- 1 lemon, sliced
- 2 tablespoons chopped fresh parsley
- 2 tablespoons chopped fresh oregano

Instructions:

1. Preheat the grill to medium-high heat.
2. Brush the sardines with olive oil.
3. Grill the sardines for 3-4 minutes per side, until cooked through.
4. Remove from the grill and drizzle with lemon juice.
5. Sprinkle with fresh parsley and oregano before serving.

Nutrition Info (per serving):

- Calories: 180
- Protein: 25g
- Carbohydrates: 2g
- Dietary Fiber: 1g
- Sugars: 0g
- Fat: 8g
- Saturated Fat: 1.5g
- Sodium: 100mg

Serves: 4

Cooking Time: 10 minute

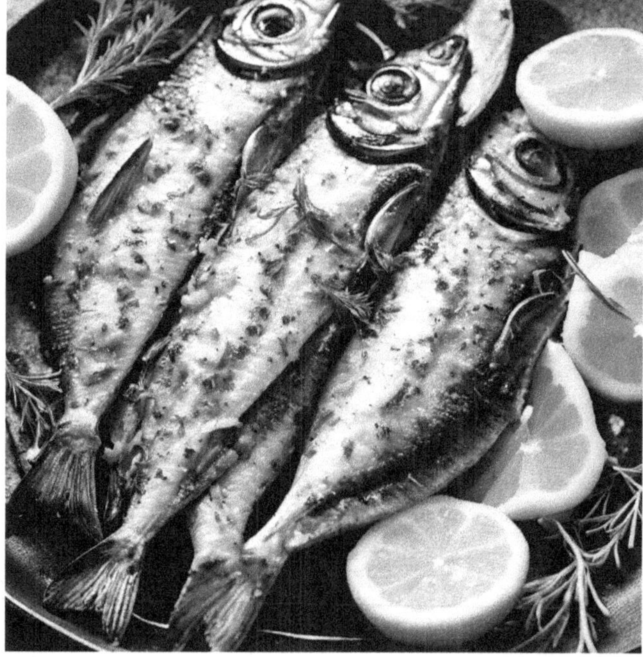

24. Paprika Baked Haddock

Ingredients:

- 4 haddock fillets
- 2 tablespoons olive oil
- 1 teaspoon paprika
- 1/2 teaspoon garlic powder
- 1 lemon, juiced

Instructions:

1. Preheat the oven to 400°F (200°C).
2. In a small bowl, mix together olive oil, paprika, and garlic powder.
3. Brush the mixture onto both sides of the haddock fillets.
4. Place the fillets on a baking sheet and bake for 12-15 minutes until the fish is opaque and flakes easily.
5. Drizzle with lemon juice before serving.

Nutrition Info (per serving):

- Calories: 180
- Protein: 28g
- Carbohydrates: 2g
- Dietary Fiber: 1g
- Sugars: 0g
- Fat: 6g
- Saturated Fat: 0.5g
- Sodium: 150mg

Serves: 4

Cooking Time: 20 minutes

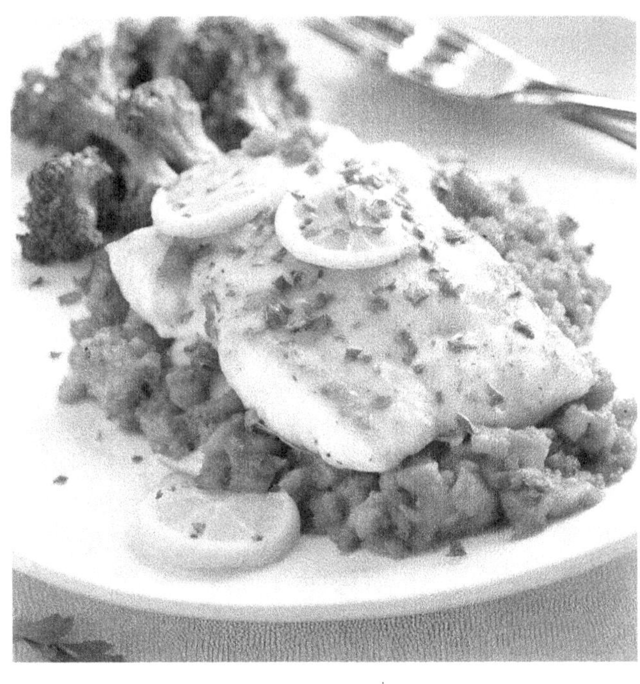

Poultry Recipes

1. Pulled Chicken Tacos

Ingredients:

- 4 boneless, skinless chicken breasts
- 1 cup chicken broth
- 1 tablespoon olive oil
- 1 tablespoon chili powder
- 1 teaspoon cumin
- 1 teaspoon garlic powder
- 1/2 teaspoon smoked paprika
- 1/2 cup salsa
- 8 small corn tortillas
- 1 cup shredded lettuce
- 1/2 cup diced tomatoes
- 1/4 cup chopped cilantro
- 1 lime, cut into wedges

Instructions:

1. In a slow cooker, add chicken breasts, chicken broth, olive oil, chili powder, cumin, garlic powder, and smoked paprika.
2. Cover and cook on low for 6 hours or until chicken is tender and easy to shred.
3. Remove chicken from the slow cooker and shred using two forks.
4. Stir in salsa and mix well.
5. Warm the tortillas in a dry skillet over medium heat for about 30 seconds on each side.
6. Fill each tortilla with pulled chicken, shredded lettuce, diced tomatoes, and chopped cilantro.
7. Serve with lime wedges.

Nutrition Info (per serving):

- Calories: 250
- Protein: 24g
- Carbohydrates: 20g
- Dietary Fiber: 3g
- Sugars: 3g
- Fat: 8g
- Saturated Fat: 1g
- Sodium: 300mg

Serves: 4

Cooking Time: 6 hours 10 minutes

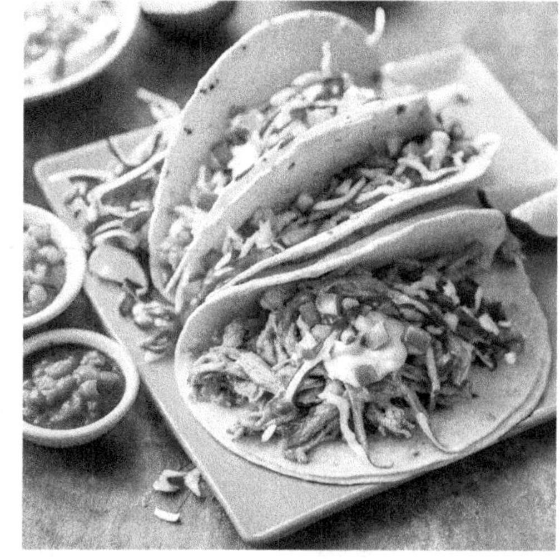

2. Turkey Stuffed Bell Peppers

Ingredients:

- 4 large bell peppers, tops cut off and seeds removed
- 1 pound ground turkey
- 1 cup cooked quinoa
- 1 cup diced tomatoes
- 1/2 cup chopped onion
- 1 cup shredded mozzarella cheese
- 1 tablespoon olive oil
- 1 teaspoon cumin
- 1 teaspoon garlic powder
- 1 teaspoon dried oregano

Instructions:

1. Preheat the oven to 375°F (190°C).
2. In a large skillet, heat olive oil over medium heat. Add chopped onion and cook until softened, about 5 minutes.
3. Add ground turkey, cumin, garlic powder, and oregano. Cook until turkey is browned and fully cooked.
4. Stir in cooked quinoa and diced tomatoes. Cook for an additional 5 minutes.
5. Stuff each bell pepper with the turkey mixture.
6. Place stuffed peppers in a baking dish and top each with shredded mozzarella cheese.
7. Cover with foil and bake for 30 minutes. Remove foil and bake for an additional 10 minutes until cheese is melted and bubbly.
8. Serve warm.

Nutrition Info (per serving):

- Calories: 350
- Protein: 30g
- Carbohydrates: 20g
- Dietary Fiber: 4g
- Sugars: 6g
- Fat: 18g
- Saturated Fat: 6g
- Sodium: 450mg

Serves: 4

Cooking Time: 50 minutes

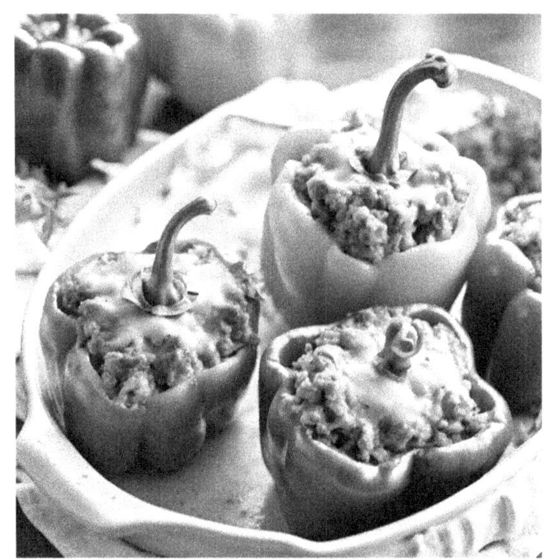

3. Turkey Spinach Meatballs

Ingredients:

- 1 pound ground turkey
- 1 cup fresh spinach, finely chopped
- 1/2 cup breadcrumbs
- 1/4 cup grated Parmesan cheese
- 1 large egg
- 1 teaspoon garlic powder
- 1 teaspoon dried basil
- 1 tablespoon olive oil

Instructions:

1. Preheat the oven to 400°F (200°C).
2. In a large bowl, combine ground turkey, spinach, breadcrumbs, Parmesan cheese, egg, garlic powder, and dried basil. Mix well.
3. Form the mixture into small meatballs and place them on a baking sheet lined with parchment paper.
4. Drizzle olive oil over the meatballs.
5. Bake for 20-25 minutes, until the meatballs are cooked through and golden brown.
6. Serve warm.

Nutrition Info (per serving):

- Calories: 220
- Protein: 25g
- Carbohydrates: 8g
- Dietary Fiber: 1g
- Sugars: 1g
- Fat: 10g
- Saturated Fat: 2g
- Sodium: 300mg

Serves: 4

Cooking Time: 30 minutes

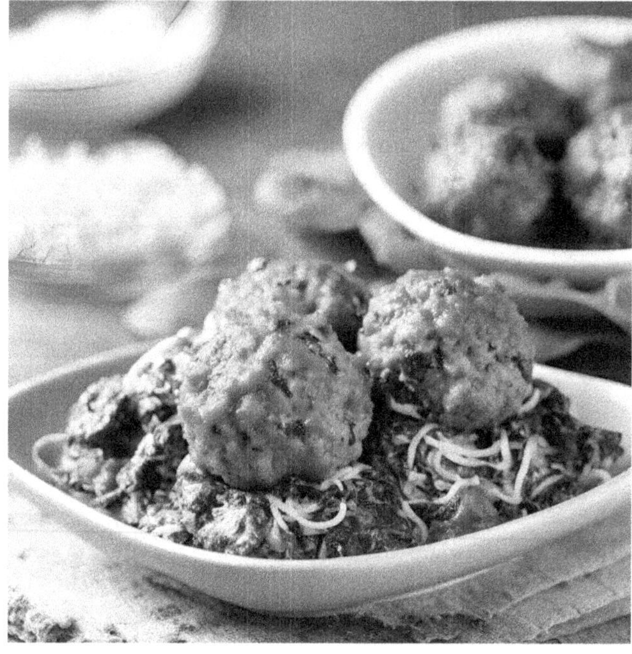

4. Chicken, Kale, and Sweet Potato Bake

Ingredients:

- 4 boneless, skinless chicken breasts
- 2 large sweet potatoes, peeled and diced
- 4 cups kale, chopped
- 2 tablespoons olive oil
- 1 teaspoon smoked paprika
- 1 teaspoon garlic powder
- 1 teaspoon dried thyme
- 1/2 cup chicken broth

Instructions:

1. Preheat the oven to 375°F (190°C).
2. In a large baking dish, combine diced sweet potatoes and chopped kale.
3. Drizzle with 1 tablespoon olive oil, and sprinkle with smoked paprika, garlic powder, and dried thyme. Toss to coat evenly.
4. Place the chicken breasts on top of the vegetable mixture and drizzle with the remaining olive oil.
5. Pour chicken broth over the vegetables.
6. Cover with foil and bake for 30 minutes. Remove foil and bake for an additional 10-15 minutes until the chicken is cooked through and the sweet potatoes are tender.
7. Serve warm.

Nutrition Info (per serving):

- Calories: 300
- Protein: 30g
- Carbohydrates: 25g
- Dietary Fiber: 5g
- Sugars: 7g
- Fat: 10g
- Saturated Fat: 1.5g
- Sodium: 300mg

Serves: 4

Cooking Time: 45 minutes

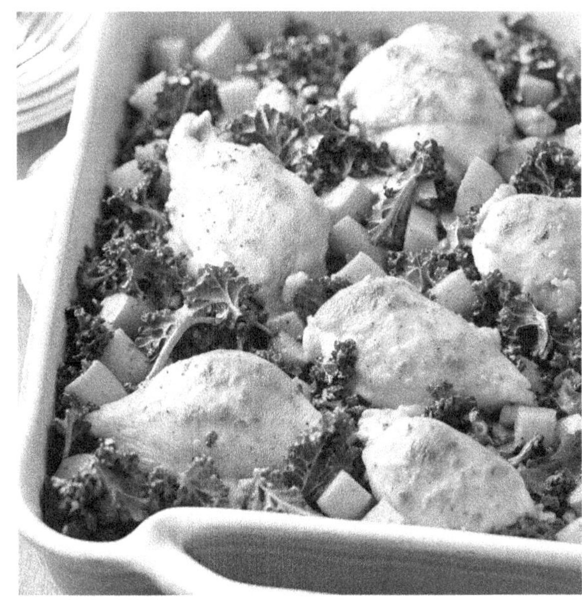

5. Slow Cooker Moroccan Chicken

Ingredients:

- 4 boneless, skinless chicken thighs
- 1 can (15 oz) chickpeas, drained and rinsed
- 1 cup diced tomatoes
- 1/2 cup dried apricots, chopped
- 1/2 cup chicken broth
- 1 tablespoon olive oil
- 1 tablespoon honey
- 1 teaspoon ground cumin
- 1 teaspoon ground cinnamon
- 1 teaspoon ground ginger
- 1/4 teaspoon turmeric

Instructions:

1. In a slow cooker, combine chicken thighs, chickpeas, diced tomatoes, dried apricots, and chicken broth.
2. In a small bowl, mix olive oil, honey, ground cumin, ground cinnamon, ground ginger, and turmeric. Pour over the chicken mixture in the slow cooker.
3. Cover and cook on low for 6-8 hours, until the chicken is tender and the flavors are well blended.
4. Serve over couscous or rice if desired.

Nutrition Info (per serving):

- Calories: 350
- Protein: 28g
- Carbohydrates: 40g
- Dietary Fiber: 8g
- Sugars: 15g
- Fat: 10g
- Saturated Fat: 2g
- Sodium: 400mg

Serves: 4

Cooking Time: 6-8 hours

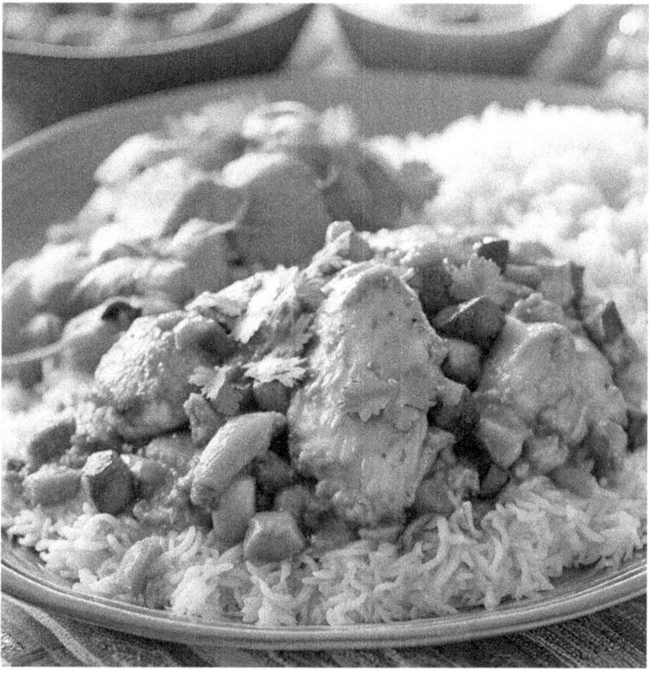

6. Chicken and Mushroom Casserole

Ingredients:

- 4 boneless, skinless chicken breasts, cut into bite-sized pieces
- 2 cups sliced mushrooms
- 1 onion, chopped
- 2 cloves garlic, minced
- 1 cup low-sodium chicken broth
- 1/2 cup unsweetened almond milk
- 2 tablespoons olive oil
- 1 tablespoon whole wheat flour
- 1 teaspoon dried thyme
- 1 teaspoon paprika

Instructions:

1. Preheat the oven to 375°F (190°C).
2. In a large skillet, heat olive oil over medium heat. Add chicken pieces and cook until browned, about 5-7 minutes.
3. Remove chicken and set aside. In the same skillet, add mushrooms, onion, and garlic. Cook until vegetables are softened, about 5 minutes.
4. Sprinkle flour over the vegetables and stir well.
5. Gradually add chicken broth and almond milk, stirring constantly until the mixture thickens.
6. Stir in thyme and paprika.
7. Return chicken to the skillet and mix well.
8. Transfer the mixture to a baking dish and bake for 20 minutes until bubbly.
9. Serve warm.

Nutrition Info (per serving):

- Calories: 280
- Protein: 30g
- Carbohydrates: 10g
- Dietary Fiber: 2g
- Sugars: 3g
- Fat: 12g
- Saturated Fat: 2g
- Sodium: 180mg

Serves: 4

Cooking Time: 40 minutes

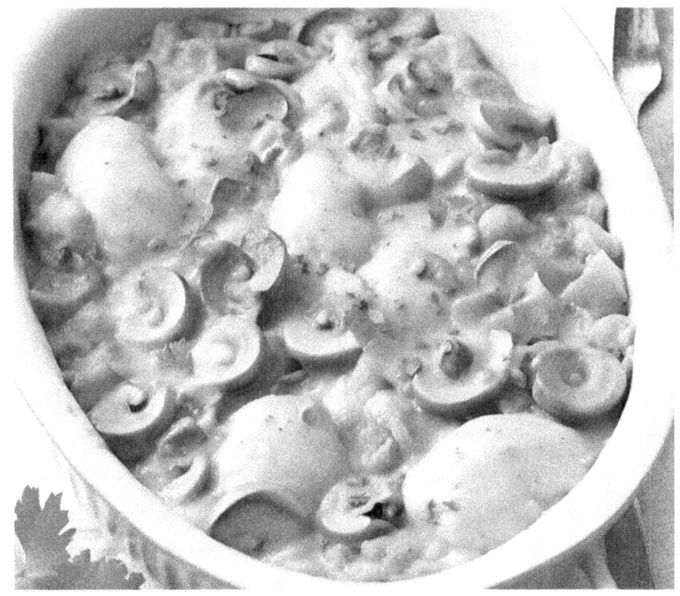

7. Turkey Chili

Ingredients:

- 1 pound ground turkey
- 1 onion, chopped
- 2 cloves garlic, minced
- 1 bell pepper, chopped
- 1 can (15 oz) black beans, drained and rinsed
- 1 can (15 oz) diced tomatoes
- 1 cup low-sodium chicken broth
- 1 tablespoon olive oil
- 1 tablespoon chili powder
- 1 teaspoon cumin
- 1 teaspoon smoked paprika
- 1/2 teaspoon oregano

Instructions:

1. In a large pot, heat olive oil over medium heat. Add ground turkey and cook until browned, about 5-7 minutes.
2. Add onion, garlic, and bell pepper. Cook until vegetables are softened, about 5 minutes.
3. Stir in chili powder, cumin, smoked paprika, and oregano. Cook for 1 minute.
4. Add black beans, diced tomatoes, and chicken broth. Bring to a simmer.
5. Reduce heat to low and cook for 30 minutes, stirring occasionally.
6. Serve warm.

Nutrition Info (per serving):

- Calories: 300
- Protein: 28g
- Carbohydrates: 25g
- Dietary Fiber: 8g
- Sugars: 5g
- Fat: 10g
- Saturated Fat: 2g
- Sodium: 400mg

Serves: 4

Cooking Time: 45 minutes

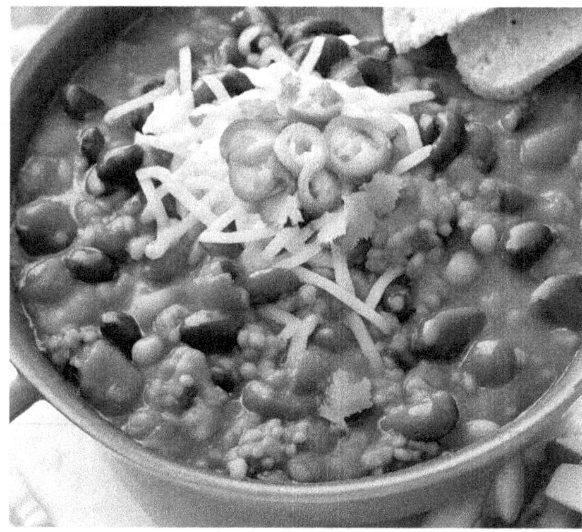

8. Lemon Chicken Orzo Soup

Ingredients:

- 2 boneless, skinless chicken breasts, diced
- 1 cup orzo pasta
- 1 onion, chopped
- 2 carrots, sliced
- 2 celery stalks, sliced
- 2 cloves garlic, minced
- 6 cups low-sodium chicken broth
- 1/4 cup lemon juice
- 1 tablespoon olive oil
- 1 teaspoon dried thyme
- 1 teaspoon dried basil

Instructions:

1. In a large pot, heat olive oil over medium heat. Add chicken and cook until browned, about 5-7 minutes.
2. Add onion, carrots, celery, and garlic. Cook until vegetables are softened, about 5 minutes.
3. Stir in chicken broth, thyme, and basil. Bring to a boil.
4. Add orzo pasta and cook until tender, about 8-10 minutes.
5. Stir in lemon juice.
6. Serve warm.

Nutrition Info (per serving):

- Calories: 260
- Protein: 24g
- Carbohydrates: 28g
- Dietary Fiber: 3g
- Sugars: 4g
- Fat: 6g
- Saturated Fat: 1g
- Sodium: 300mg

Serves: 4

Cooking Time: 30 minutes

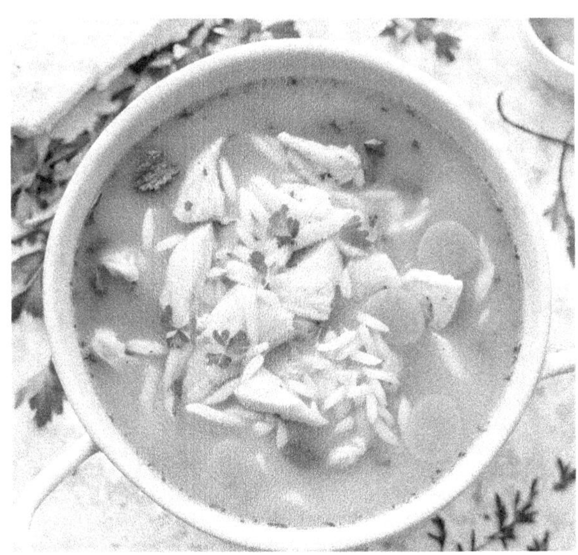

9. Chicken and Quinoa Soup

Ingredients:

- 2 boneless, skinless chicken breasts, diced
- 1 cup quinoa, rinsed
- 1 onion, chopped
- 2 carrots, sliced
- 2 celery stalks, sliced
- 2 cloves garlic, minced
- 6 cups low-sodium chicken broth
- 1 tablespoon olive oil
- 1 teaspoon dried thyme
- 1 teaspoon dried rosemary

Instructions:

1. In a large pot, heat olive oil over medium heat. Add chicken and cook until browned, about 5-7 minutes.
2. Add onion, carrots, celery, and garlic. Cook until vegetables are softened, about 5 minutes.
3. Stir in chicken broth, quinoa, thyme, and rosemary. Bring to a boil.
4. Reduce heat to low and simmer for 20 minutes, until quinoa is cooked and chicken is tender.
5. Serve warm.

Nutrition Info (per serving):

- Calories: 280
- Protein: 25g
- Carbohydrates: 28g
- Dietary Fiber: 4g
- Sugars: 4g
- Fat: 7g
- Saturated Fat: 1g
- Sodium: 250mg

Serves: 4

Cooking Time: 35 minutes

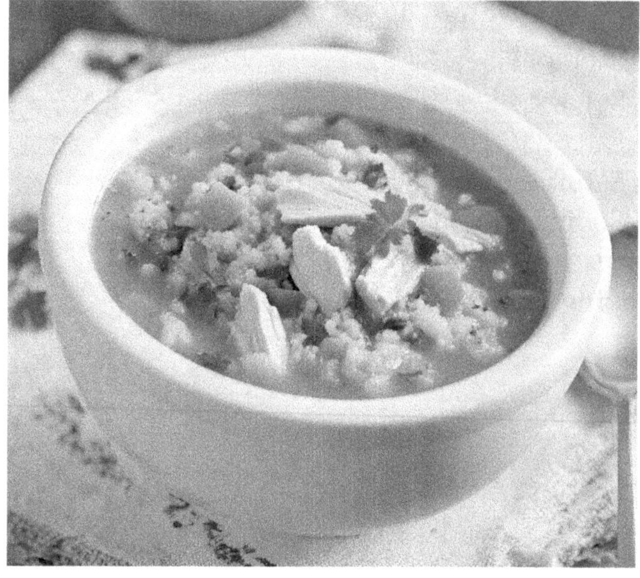

10. Turkey and Sweet Potato Stew

Ingredients:

- 1 pound ground turkey
- 2 large sweet potatoes, peeled and diced
- 1 onion, chopped
- 2 carrots, sliced
- 2 cloves garlic, minced
- 4 cups low-sodium chicken broth
- 1 can (15 oz) diced tomatoes
- 1 tablespoon olive oil
- 1 teaspoon ground cumin
- 1 teaspoon smoked paprika
- 1 teaspoon dried thyme

Instructions:

1. In a large pot, heat olive oil over medium heat. Add ground turkey and cook until browned, about 5-7 minutes.
2. Add onion, carrots, and garlic. Cook until vegetables are softened, about 5 minutes.
3. Stir in sweet potatoes, chicken broth, diced tomatoes, cumin, smoked paprika, and thyme. Bring to a boil.
4. Reduce heat to low and simmer for 25-30 minutes, until sweet potatoes are tender.
5. Serve warm.

Nutrition Info (per serving):

- Calories: 350
- Protein: 25g
- Carbohydrates: 40g
- Dietary Fiber: 6g
- Sugars: 10g
- Fat: 10g
- Saturated Fat: 2g
- Sodium: 300mg

Serves: 4

Cooking Time: 45 minutes

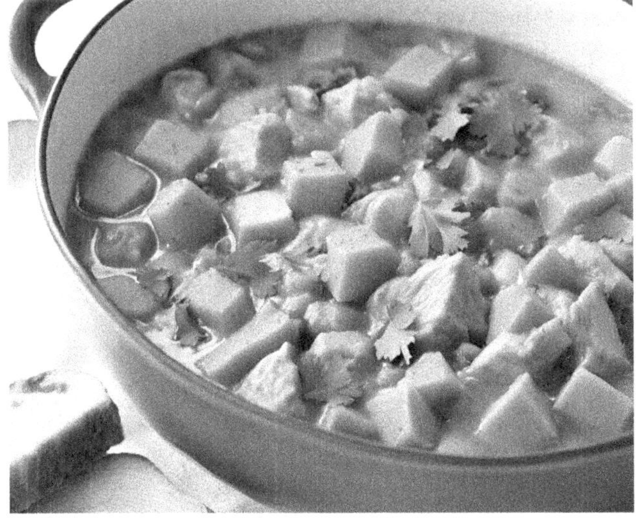

11. Chicken Vegetable Soup

Ingredients:

- 2 boneless, skinless chicken breasts, diced
- 1 onion, chopped
- 2 carrots, sliced
- 2 celery stalks, sliced
- 2 cups green beans, chopped
- 2 cloves garlic, minced
- 6 cups low-sodium chicken broth
- 1 can (15 oz) diced tomatoes
- 1 tablespoon olive oil
- 1 teaspoon dried basil
- 1 teaspoon dried oregano

Instructions:

1. In a large pot, heat olive oil over medium heat. Add chicken and cook until browned, about 5-7 minutes.
2. Add onion, carrots, celery, green beans, and garlic. Cook until vegetables are softened, about 5 minutes.
3. Stir in chicken broth, diced tomatoes, basil, and oregano. Bring to a boil.
4. Reduce heat to low and simmer for 20 minutes, until chicken is cooked and vegetables are tender.
5. Serve warm.

Nutrition Info (per serving):

- Calories: 250
- Protein: 24g
- Carbohydrates: 20g
- Dietary Fiber: 5g
- Sugars: 8g
- Fat: 8g
- Saturated Fat: 1g
- Sodium: 280mg

Serves: 4

Cooking Time: 30 minutes

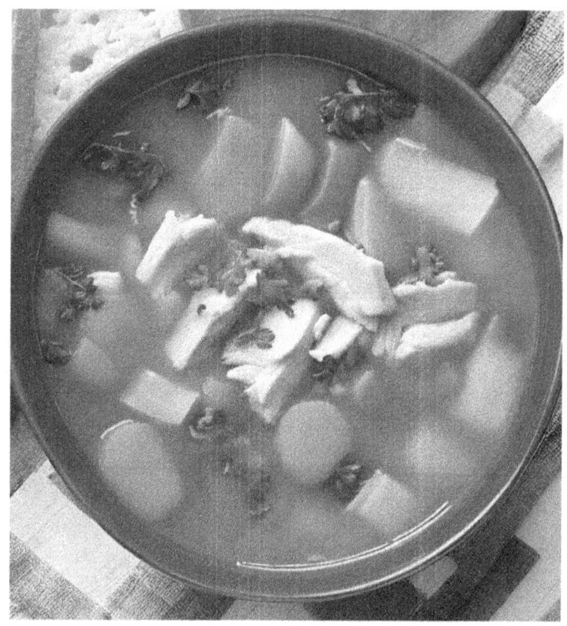

12. Chicken Piccata

Ingredients:

- 4 boneless, skinless chicken breasts, pounded thin
- 1/4 cup whole wheat flour
- 1/4 cup lemon juice
- 1/2 cup low-sodium chicken broth
- 1/4 cup capers, drained
- 2 tablespoons olive oil
- 1 tablespoon chopped fresh parsley

Instructions:

1. Dredge the chicken breasts in whole wheat flour, shaking off excess.
2. In a large skillet, heat olive oil over medium-high heat. Add chicken and cook until browned, about 3-4 minutes per side.
3. Remove chicken from the skillet and set aside.
4. In the same skillet, add lemon juice, chicken broth, and capers. Bring to a simmer and cook for 2 minutes.
5. Return chicken to the skillet and cook for an additional 5 minutes, until cooked through and sauce has thickened.
6. Garnish with chopped fresh parsley before serving.

Nutrition Info (per serving):

- Calories: 280
- Protein: 30g
- Carbohydrates: 10g
- Dietary Fiber: 2g
- Sugars: 2g
- Fat: 12g
- Saturated Fat: 2g
- Sodium: 350mg

Serves: 4

Cooking Time: 20 minutes

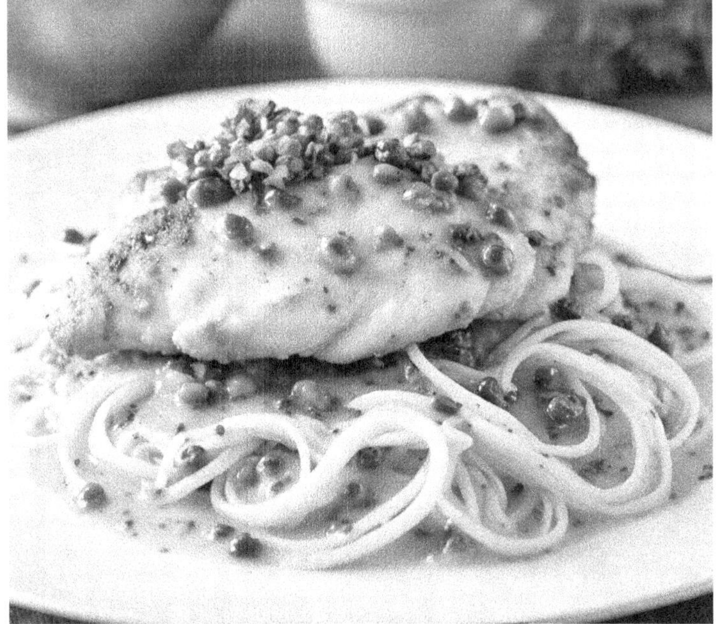

13. Herb Grilled Turkey Steaks

Ingredients:

- 4 turkey steaks
- 1/4 cup olive oil
- 2 tablespoons lemon juice
- 1 tablespoon chopped fresh rosemary
- 1 tablespoon chopped fresh thyme
- 1 tablespoon chopped fresh parsley
- 2 cloves garlic, minced

Instructions:

1. In a small bowl, whisk together olive oil, lemon juice, rosemary, thyme, parsley, and garlic.
2. Brush the mixture onto both sides of the turkey steaks.
3. Preheat the grill to medium-high heat.
4. Grill the turkey steaks for 5-7 minutes per side, until cooked through and nicely charred.
5. Serve immediately.

Nutrition Info (per serving):

- Calories: 250
- Protein: 32g
- Carbohydrates: 2g
- Dietary Fiber: 0g
- Sugars: 0g
- Fat: 12g
- Saturated Fat: 2g
- Sodium: 80mg

Serves: 4

Cooking Time: 15 minutes

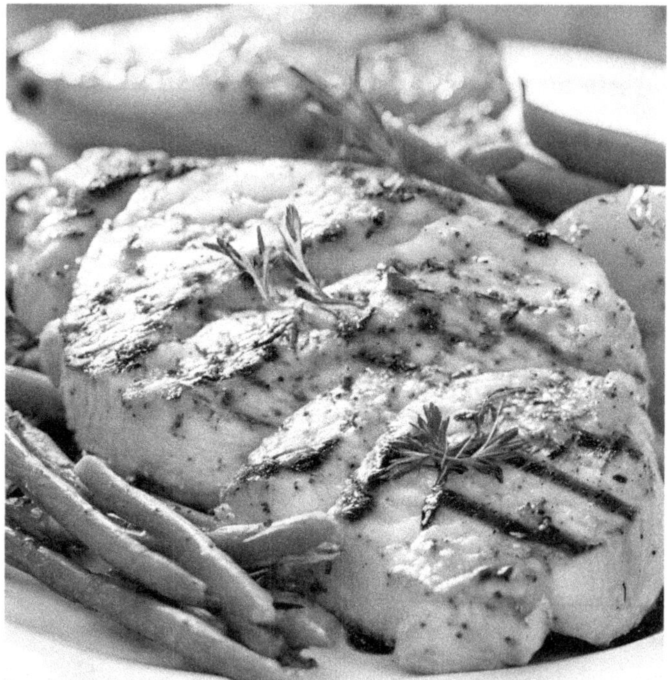

14. Smoky Paprika Chicken

Ingredients:

- 4 boneless, skinless chicken breasts
- 2 tablespoons olive oil
- 2 teaspoons smoked paprika
- 1 teaspoon garlic powder
- 1 teaspoon dried oregano
- 1 tablespoon lemon juice

Instructions:

1. Preheat the oven to 375°F (190°C).
2. In a small bowl, mix together olive oil, smoked paprika, garlic powder, dried oregano, and lemon juice.
3. Brush the mixture onto both sides of the chicken breasts.
4. Place the chicken breasts on a baking sheet.
5. Bake for 25-30 minutes, until the chicken is cooked through and juices run clear.
6. Serve immediately.

Nutrition Info (per serving):

- Calories: 220
- Protein: 28g
- Carbohydrates: 2g
- Dietary Fiber: 1g
- Sugars: 0g
- Fat: 10g
- Saturated Fat: 1.5g
- Sodium: 90mg

Serves: 4

Cooking Time: 35 minutes

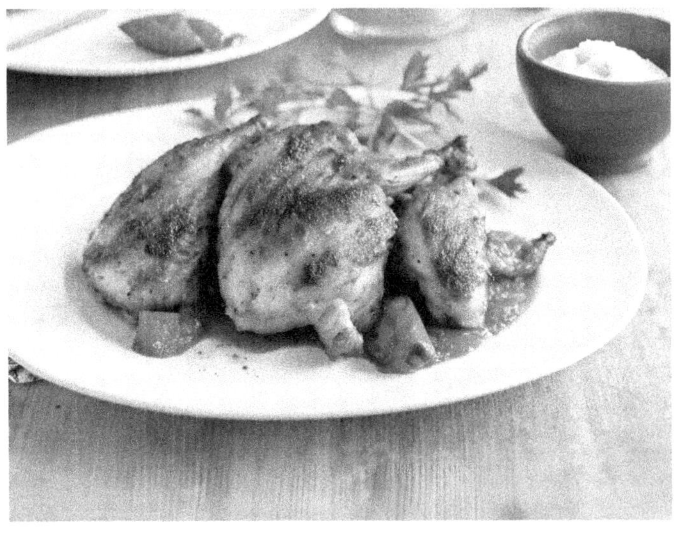

15. Chicken and Vegetable Kabobs

Ingredients:

- 4 boneless, skinless chicken breasts, cut into chunks
- 2 bell peppers, cut into chunks
- 1 red onion, cut into chunks
- 1 zucchini, sliced
- 1/4 cup olive oil
- 1 tablespoon lemon juice
- 1 teaspoon dried basil
- 1 teaspoon garlic powder

Instructions:

1. Preheat the grill to medium-high heat.
2. In a small bowl, whisk together olive oil, lemon juice, dried basil, and garlic powder.
3. Thread chicken, bell peppers, red onion, and zucchini onto skewers.
4. Brush the olive oil mixture onto the skewers.
5. Grill the kabobs for 10-12 minutes, turning occasionally, until the chicken is cooked through and vegetables are tender.
6. Serve immediately.

Nutrition Info (per serving):

- Calories: 250
- Protein: 28g
- Carbohydrates: 8g
- Dietary Fiber: 2g
- Sugars: 4g
- Fat: 12g
- Saturated Fat: 2g
- Sodium: 80mg

Serves: 4
Cooking Time: 20 minutes

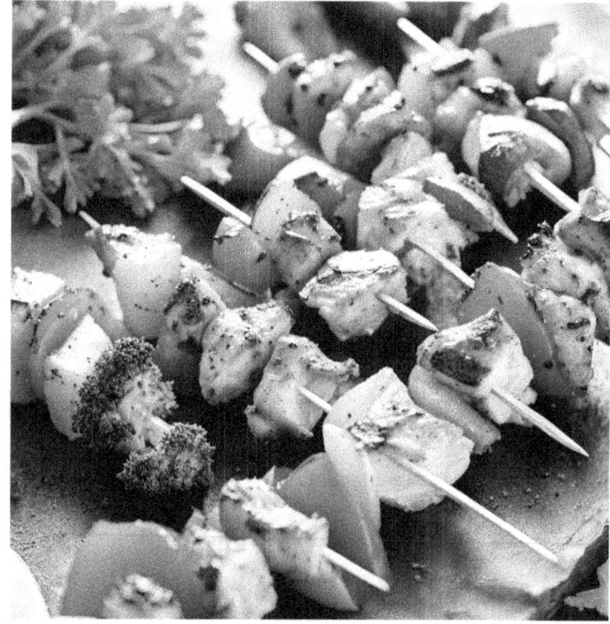

16. Honey Mustard Chicken Salad

Ingredients:

- 4 boneless, skinless chicken breasts
- 1/4 cup honey
- 1/4 cup Dijon mustard
- 2 tablespoons olive oil
- 1 tablespoon lemon juice
- 6 cups mixed salad greens
- 1/2 cup cherry tomatoes, halved
- 1/4 cup sliced almonds

Instructions:

1. Preheat the grill to medium-high heat.
2. In a small bowl, whisk together honey, Dijon mustard, olive oil, and lemon juice.
3. Brush the mixture onto both sides of the chicken breasts.
4. Grill the chicken for 5-7 minutes per side, until cooked through and nicely charred.
5. Let the chicken rest for a few minutes, then slice into strips.
6. In a large bowl, toss mixed salad greens, cherry tomatoes, and sliced almonds.
7. Top with grilled chicken strips and drizzle with any remaining honey mustard mixture.
8. Serve immediately.

Nutrition Info (per serving):

- Calories: 320
- Protein: 30g
- Carbohydrates: 15g
- Dietary Fiber: 3g
- Sugars: 12g
- Fat: 15g
- Saturated Fat: 2.5g
- Sodium: 150mg

Serves: 4

Cooking Time: 20 minutes

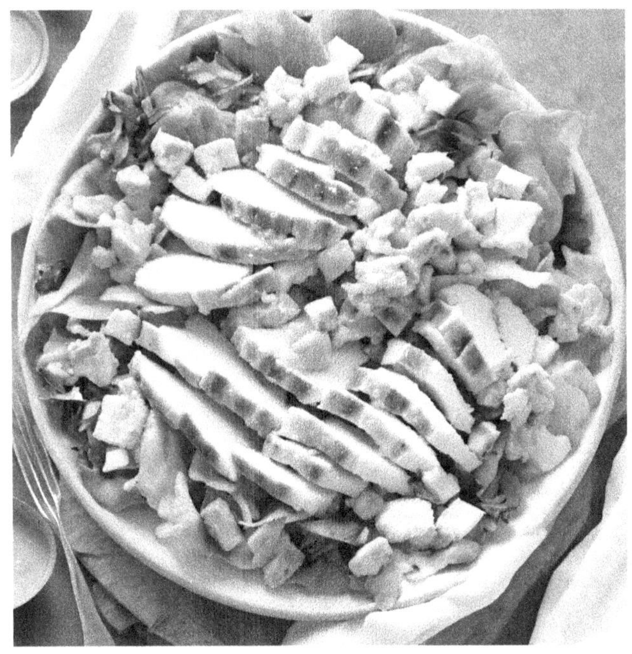

17. Chicken Caesar Salad

Ingredients:

- 4 boneless, skinless chicken breasts
- 1 tablespoon olive oil
- 6 cups Romaine lettuce, chopped
- 1/2 cup grated Parmesan cheese
- 1 cup croutons
- 1/4 cup Caesar dressing

Instructions:

1. Preheat the grill to medium-high heat.
2. Brush the chicken breasts with olive oil.
3. Grill the chicken for 5-7 minutes per side, until cooked through and nicely charred.
4. Let the chicken rest for a few minutes, then slice into strips.
5. In a large bowl, toss Romaine lettuce with Caesar dressing.
6. Top with grilled chicken strips, Parmesan cheese, and croutons.
7. Serve immediately.

Nutrition Info (per serving):

- Calories: 350
- Protein: 32g
- Carbohydrates: 12g
- Dietary Fiber: 3g
- Sugars: 2g
- Fat: 20g
- Saturated Fat: 5g
- Sodium: 450mg

Serves: 4

Cooking Time: 20 minutes

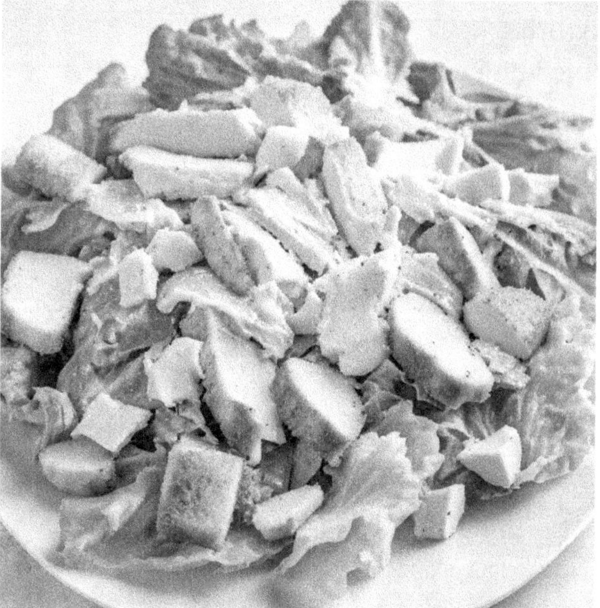

18. Greek Lemon Chicken Skewers

Ingredients:

- 4 boneless, skinless chicken breasts, cut into chunks
- 1/4 cup olive oil
- 2 tablespoons lemon juice
- 1 tablespoon chopped fresh oregano
- 1 teaspoon garlic powder

Instructions:

1. Preheat the grill to medium-high heat.
2. In a small bowl, whisk together olive oil, lemon juice, oregano, and garlic powder.
3. Thread the chicken chunks onto skewers.
4. Brush the olive oil mixture onto the skewers.
5. Grill the skewers for 10-12 minutes, turning occasionally, until the chicken is cooked through and nicely charred.
6. Serve immediately.

Nutrition Info (per serving):

- Calories: 250
- Protein: 28g
- Carbohydrates: 2g
- Dietary Fiber: 0g
- Sugars: 0g
- Fat: 12g
- Saturated Fat: 2g
- Sodium: 80mg

Serves: 4

Cooking Time: 20 minutes

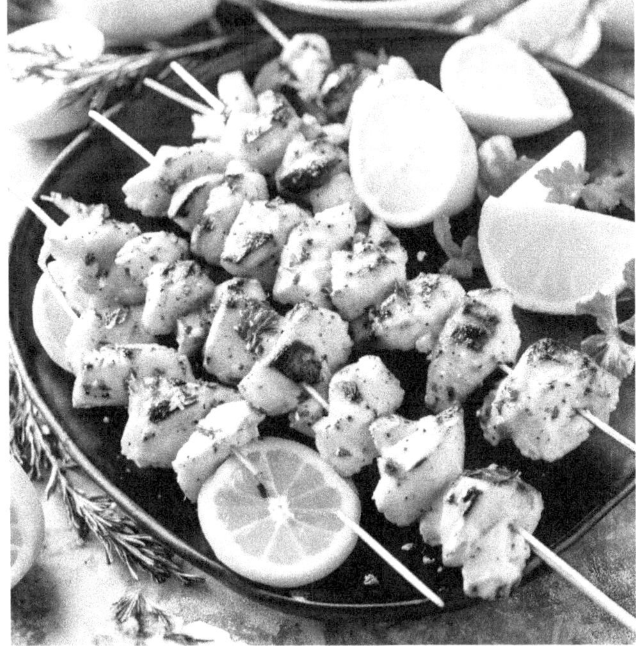

19. Orange and Thyme Chicken

Ingredients:

- 4 boneless, skinless chicken breasts
- 1/4 cup orange juice
- 1 tablespoon olive oil
- 1 tablespoon chopped fresh thyme
- 1 teaspoon garlic powder

Instructions:

1. Preheat the oven to 375°F (190°C).
2. In a small bowl, mix together orange juice, olive oil, thyme, and garlic powder.
3. Brush the mixture onto both sides of the chicken breasts.
4. Place the chicken breasts on a baking sheet.
5. Bake for 25-30 minutes, until the chicken is cooked through and juices run clear.
6. Serve immediately.

Nutrition Info (per serving):

- Calories: 220
- Protein: 28g
- Carbohydrates: 3g
- Dietary Fiber: 1g
- Sugars: 2g
- Fat: 10g
- Saturated Fat: 1.5g
- Sodium: 80mg

Serves: 4

Cooking Time: 35 minutes

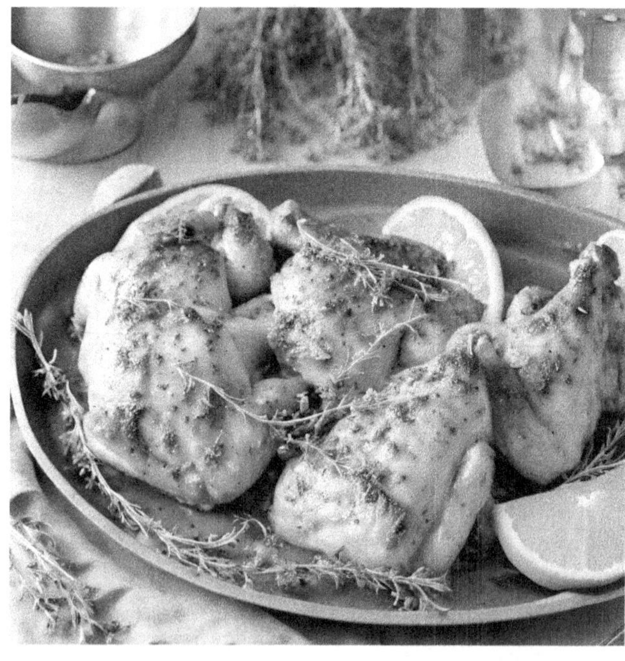

20. Garlic Herb Turkey Patties

Ingredients:

- 1 pound ground turkey
- 2 cloves garlic, minced
- 1 tablespoon chopped fresh parsley
- 1 tablespoon chopped fresh basil
- 1 teaspoon dried oregano
- 1 tablespoon olive oil

Instructions:

1. In a large bowl, combine ground turkey, garlic, parsley, basil, and oregano. Mix well.
2. Form the mixture into patties.
3. Heat olive oil in a large skillet over medium heat.
4. Cook the patties for 5-7 minutes per side, until cooked through and browned.
5. Serve immediately.

Nutrition Info (per serving):

- Calories: 220
- Protein: 26g
- Carbohydrates: 2g
- Dietary Fiber: 0g
- Sugars: 0g
- Fat: 12g
- Saturated Fat: 2g
- Sodium: 80mg

Serves: 4

Cooking Time: 20 minutes

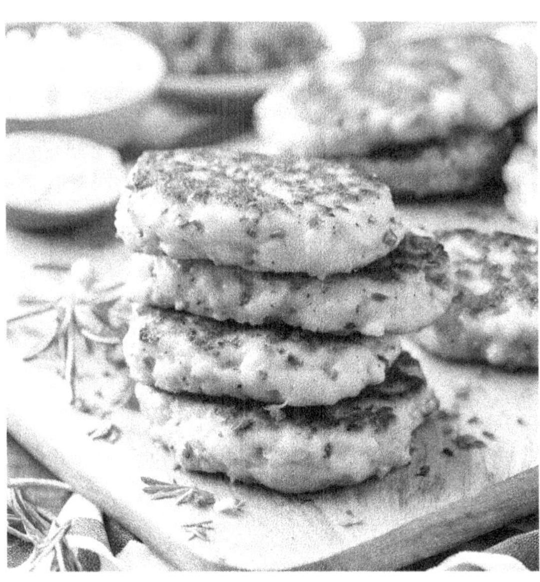

21. Mediterranean Stuffed Chicken

Ingredients:

- 4 boneless, skinless chicken breasts
- 1/2 cup chopped spinach
- 1/4 cup sun-dried tomatoes, chopped
- 1/4 cup crumbled feta cheese
- 1 tablespoon olive oil
- 1 teaspoon dried oregano

Instructions:

1. Preheat the oven to 375°F (190°C).
2. In a small bowl, mix together spinach, sun-dried tomatoes, and feta cheese.
3. Cut a pocket into each chicken breast and stuff with the spinach mixture.
4. Secure with toothpicks.
5. Brush the chicken breasts with olive oil and sprinkle with dried oregano.
6. Place the chicken breasts on a baking sheet.
7. Bake for 25-30 minutes, until the chicken is cooked through and juices run clear.
8. Serve immediately.

Nutrition Info (per serving):

- Calories: 280
- Protein: 30g
- Carbohydrates: 4g
- Dietary Fiber: 1g
- Sugars: 2g
- Fat: 14g
- Saturated Fat: 4g
- Sodium: 250mg

Serves: 4

Cooking Time: 35 minutes

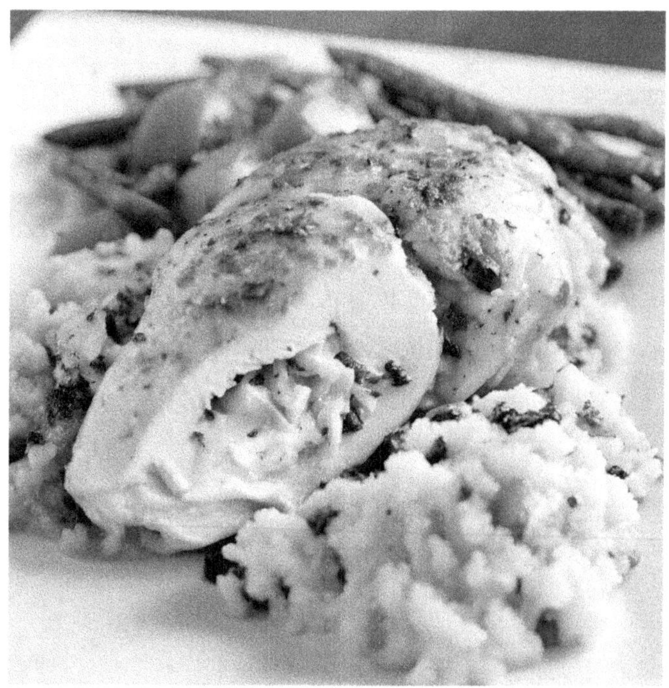

22. Spiced Roast Turkey

Ingredients:

- 1 whole turkey (about 12 pounds)
- 1/4 cup olive oil
- 1 tablespoon smoked paprika
- 1 tablespoon garlic powder
- 1 teaspoon ground cumin
- 1 teaspoon dried thyme

Instructions:

1. Preheat the oven to 325°F (165°C).
2. In a small bowl, mix together olive oil, smoked paprika, garlic powder, cumin, and thyme.
3. Rub the mixture all over the turkey.
4. Place the turkey on a roasting rack in a roasting pan.
5. Roast the turkey for 3-3.5 hours, until the internal temperature reaches 165°F (75°C).
6. Let the turkey rest for 20 minutes before carving.
7. Serve immediately.

Nutrition Info (per serving):

- Calories: 320
- Protein: 45g
- Carbohydrates: 2g
- Dietary Fiber: 1g
- Sugars: 0g
- Fat: 14g
- Saturated Fat: 3g
- Sodium: 90mg

Serves: 10
Cooking Time: 3.5 hours

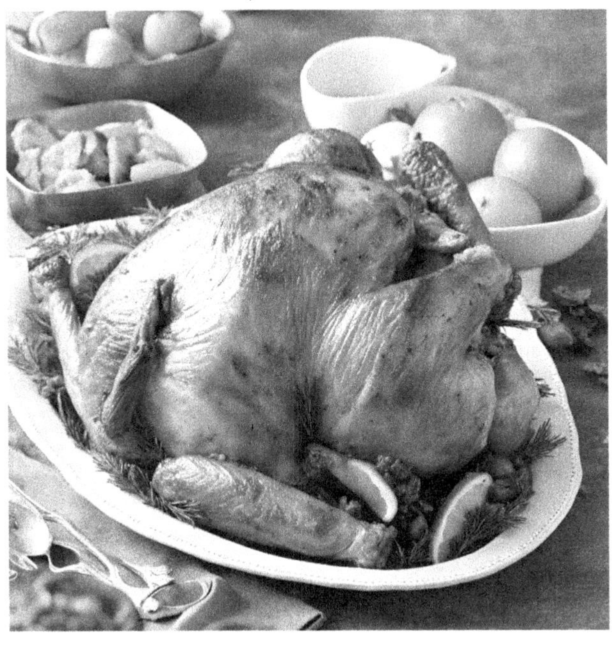

23. Rosemary Chicken and Potatoes

Ingredients:

- 4 boneless, skinless chicken breasts
- 4 cups baby potatoes, halved
- 2 tablespoons olive oil
- 2 tablespoons chopped fresh rosemary
- 1 teaspoon garlic powder
- 1/4 cup lemon juice

Instructions:

1. Preheat the oven to 400°F (200°C).
2. In a large bowl, toss baby potatoes with 1 tablespoon olive oil, half the chopped rosemary, and garlic powder.
3. Spread the potatoes on a baking sheet and roast for 15 minutes.
4. Meanwhile, brush the chicken breasts with remaining olive oil and sprinkle with the remaining rosemary.
5. After 15 minutes, add the chicken breasts to the baking sheet with the potatoes.
6. Drizzle lemon juice over the chicken and potatoes.
7. Roast for an additional 20-25 minutes, until the chicken is cooked through and potatoes are tender.
8. Serve immediately.

Nutrition Info (per serving):

- Calories: 350
- Protein: 30g
- Carbohydrates: 30g
- Dietary Fiber: 4g
- Sugars: 2g
- Fat: 14g
- Saturated Fat: 2.5g
- Sodium: 120mg

Serves: 4

Cooking Time: 40 minutes

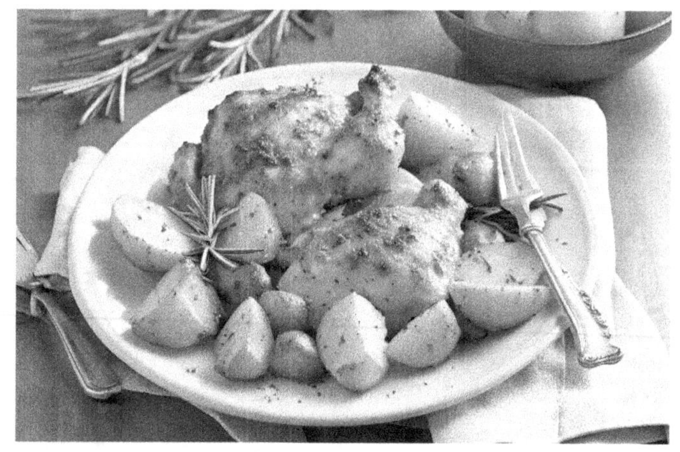

Snacks & Sides Recipes

1. Kale Chips

Ingredients:
- 1 bunch kale, stems removed and leaves torn into bite-sized pieces
- 1 tablespoon olive oil
- 1 teaspoon smoked paprika

Instructions:
1. Preheat the oven to 300°F (150°C).
2. In a large bowl, toss the kale leaves with olive oil and smoked paprika until evenly coated.
3. Spread the kale leaves in a single layer on a baking sheet.
4. Bake for 20-25 minutes, until the edges are crisp but not burnt.
5. Allow to cool before serving.

Nutrition Info (per serving):
- Calories: 70
- Protein: 3g
- Carbohydrates: 7g
- Dietary Fiber: 2g
- Sugars: 1g
- Fat: 4g
- Saturated Fat: 0.5g
- Sodium: 30mg

Serves: 4
Cooking Time: 30 minutes

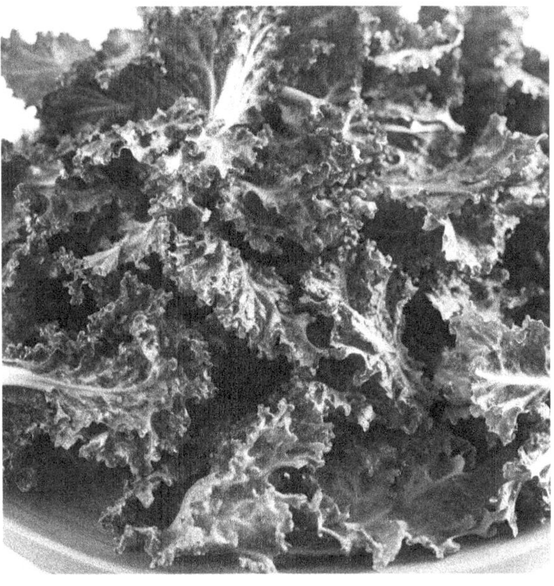

2. Edamame with Sea Salt

Ingredients:

- 2 cups edamame (in pods)
- 1 teaspoon sea salt

Instructions:

1. Bring a pot of water to a boil.
2. Add the edamame and cook for 3-5 minutes, until tender.
3. Drain the edamame and sprinkle with sea salt.
4. Serve warm or at room temperature.

Nutrition Info (per serving):

- Calories: 120
- Protein: 10g
- Carbohydrates: 10g
- Dietary Fiber: 4g
- Sugars: 1g
- Fat: 4g
- Saturated Fat: 0.5g
- Sodium: 230mg

Serves: 4

Cooking Time: 10 minutes

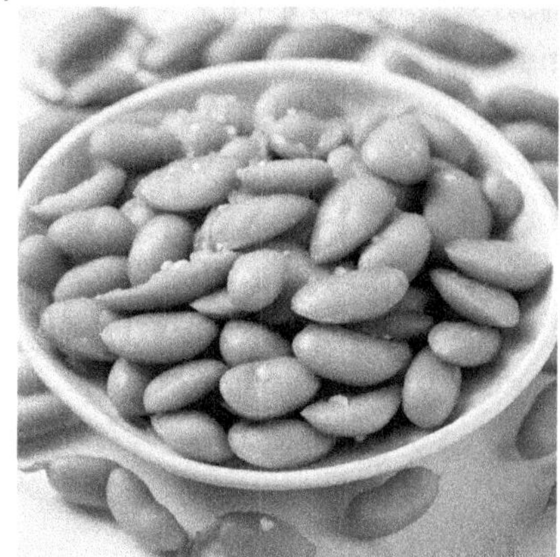

3. Almond Yogurt with Honey and Walnuts

Ingredients:

- 2 cups unsweetened almond yogurt
- 2 tablespoons honey
- 1/4 cup chopped walnuts

Instructions:

1. Divide the almond yogurt into four bowls.
2. Drizzle honey over the yogurt.
3. Sprinkle chopped walnuts on top.
4. Serve immediately.

Nutrition Info (per serving):

- Calories: 150
- Protein: 4g
- Carbohydrates: 20g
- Dietary Fiber: 2g
- Sugars: 15g
- Fat: 7g
- Saturated Fat: 0.5g
- Sodium: 50mg

Serves: 4

Cooking Time: 5 minutes

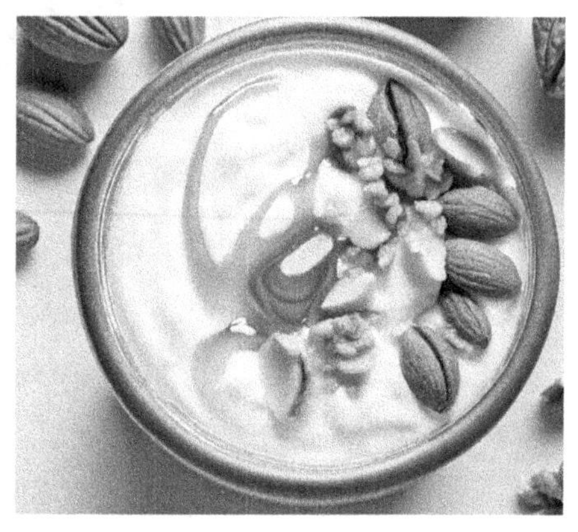

4. Carrot Sticks with Hummus

Ingredients:

- 4 large carrots, peeled and cut into sticks
- 1 cup hummus

Instructions:

1. Arrange the carrot sticks on a plate.
2. Serve with a side of hummus for dipping.

Nutrition Info (per serving):

- Calories: 100
- Protein: 3g
- Carbohydrates: 15g
- Dietary Fiber: 5g
- Sugars: 6g
- Fat: 4g
- Saturated Fat: 0.5g
- Sodium: 200mg

Serves: 4

Cooking Time: 5 minutes

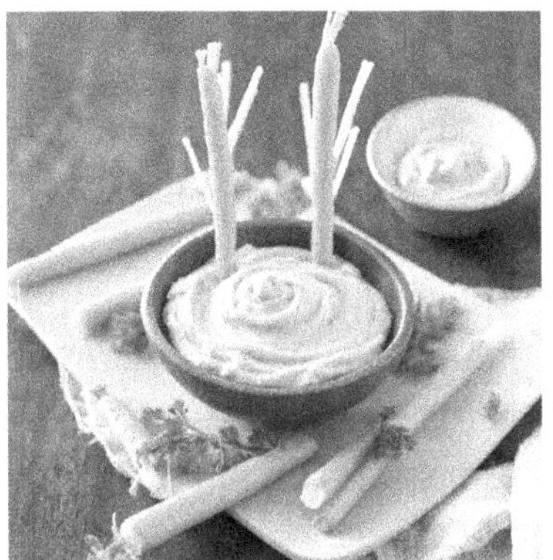

5. Calcium-Fortified Orange Juice Smoothie

Ingredients:

- 1 cup calcium-fortified orange juice
- 1/2 cup unsweetened almond milk
- 1 banana
- 1/2 cup frozen mango chunks
- 1 tablespoon chia seeds

Instructions:

1. Combine all ingredients in a blender.
2. Blend on high until smooth and creamy.
3. Pour into glasses and serve immediately.

Nutrition Info (per serving):

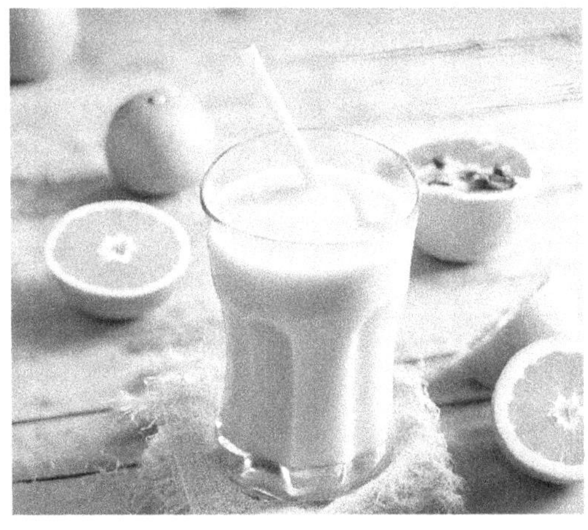

- Calories: 170
- Protein: 3g
- Carbohydrates: 35g
- Dietary Fiber: 6g
- Sugars: 20g
- Fat: 4g
- Saturated Fat: 0.5g
- Sodium: 40mg

Serves: 2

Cooking Time: 5 minutes

6. Oat Bran Muffins

Ingredients:

- 1 cup oat bran
- 1 cup whole wheat flour
- 1/4 cup brown sugar
- 1 teaspoon baking powder
- 1/2 teaspoon baking soda
- 1 teaspoon cinnamon
- 1/2 cup unsweetened applesauce
- 1 cup unsweetened almond milk
- 1 large egg
- 1 teaspoon vanilla extract

Instructions:

1. Preheat the oven to 375°F (190°C) and line a muffin tin with paper liners.
2. In a large bowl, combine oat bran, whole wheat flour, brown sugar, baking powder, baking soda, and cinnamon.
3. In another bowl, mix applesauce, almond milk, egg, and vanilla extract.
4. Add the wet ingredients to the dry ingredients and mix until just combined.
5. Divide the batter evenly among the muffin cups.
6. Bake for 15-18 minutes, until a toothpick inserted into the center comes out clean.
7. Allow to cool before serving.

Nutrition Info (per serving):

- Calories: 150
- Protein: 4g
- Carbohydrates: 28g
- Dietary Fiber: 5g
- Sugars: 8g
- Fat: 3g
- Saturated Fat: 0.5g
- Sodium: 150mg

Serves: 12

Cooking Time: 20 minutes

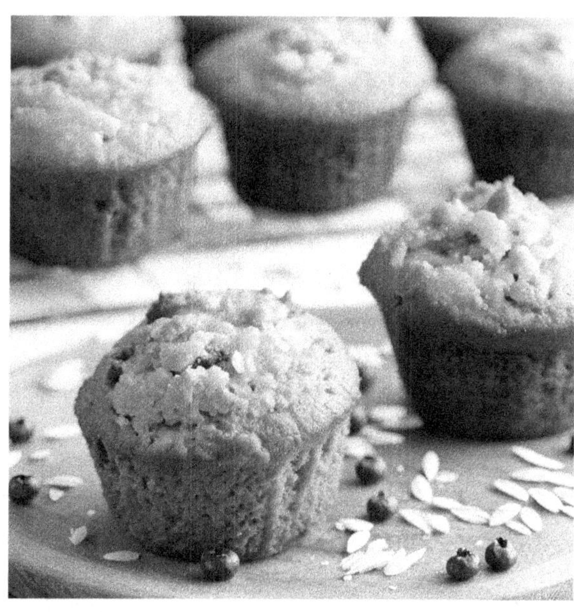

7. Roasted Chickpeas

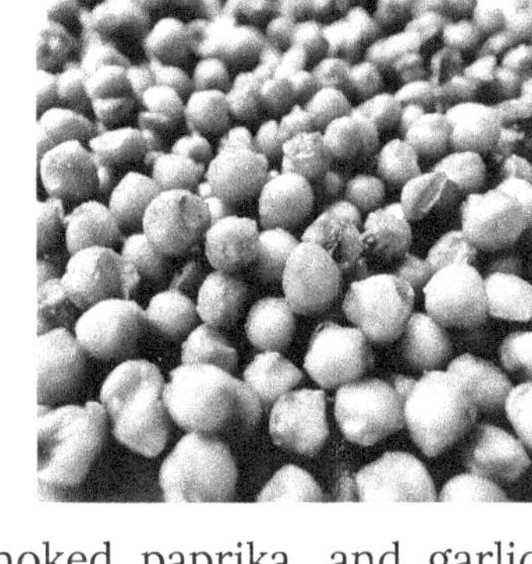

Ingredients:
- 1 can (15 oz) chickpeas, drained and rinsed
- 1 tablespoon olive oil
- 1 teaspoon smoked paprika
- 1/2 teaspoon garlic powder

Instructions:
1. Preheat the oven to 400°F (200°C).
2. Pat the chickpeas dry with a paper towel.
3. In a bowl, toss the chickpeas with olive oil, smoked paprika, and garlic powder.
4. Spread the chickpeas in a single layer on a baking sheet.
5. Roast for 20-25 minutes, stirring halfway through, until crispy.
6. Allow to cool slightly before serving.

Nutrition Info (per serving):
- Calories: 140 Protein: 6g Carbohydrates: 18g Dietary Fiber: 6g Sugars: 1g
- Fat: 5g
- Saturated Fat: 0.5g
- Sodium: 220mg

Serves: 4
Cooking Time: 30 minutes

8. Stuffed Dates with Almond Butter

Ingredients:
- 12 Medjool dates, pitted
- 1/4 cup almond butter
- 1/4 cup chopped walnuts

Instructions:
1. Carefully slice each date lengthwise to create an opening.
2. Stuff each date with about 1 teaspoon of almond butter.
3. Sprinkle chopped walnuts over the almond butter.
4. Serve immediately or store in the refrigerator until ready to eat.

Nutrition Info (per serving):
- Calories: 150 Protein: 3g Carbohydrates: 22g Dietary Fiber: 3g
- Sugars: 18g
- Fat: 7g
- Saturated Fat: 0.5g
- Sodium: 1mg

Serves: 4
Cooking Time: 10 minutes

9. Quinoa Tabbouleh

Ingredients:

- 1 cup quinoa, rinsed
- 2 cups water
- 1 cup chopped fresh parsley
- 1/2 cup chopped fresh mint
- 1 cup diced tomatoes
- 1/2 cup diced cucumber
- 1/4 cup diced red onion
- 1/4 cup lemon juice
- 1/4 cup olive oil
- 1 teaspoon garlic powder

Instructions:

1. In a me⋯⋯ce heat, and simmer ⋯⋯⋯sorbed.
2. Let the ⋯
3. In a larg⋯, cucumber, and red ⋯
4. In a sma⋯owder. Pour over the ⋯
5. Serve ch⋯

Nutrition In⋯

- Calories:
- Protein:
- Carbohy⋯
- Dietary ⋯
- Sugars: ⋯
- Fat: 10g
- Saturate⋯
- Sodium: ⋯

Serves: 4

Cooking Tim⋯ 20 minutes

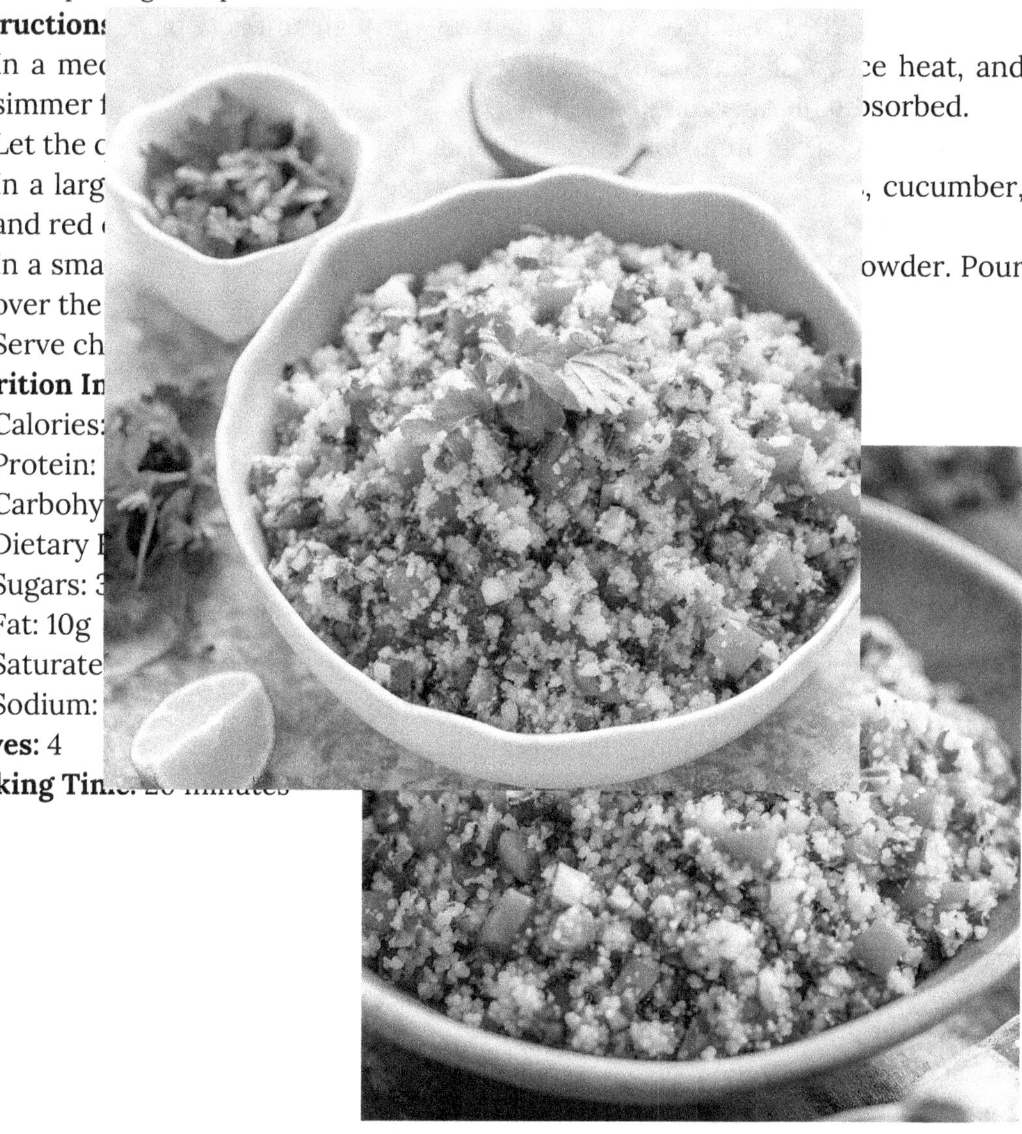

10. Steamed Broccoli with Almond Slivers

Ingredients:

- 4 cups broccoli florets
- 1 tablespoon olive oil
- 1/4 cup slivered almonds
- 1 teaspoon garlic powder

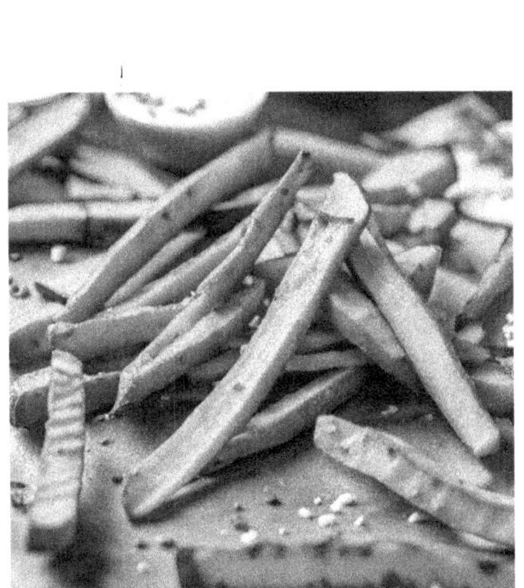

Instructions:

1. Steam the broccoli florets for 5-7 minutes, until tender but still crisp.
2. In a small skillet, heat olive oil over medium heat. Add slivered almonds and garlic powder, and sauté until the almonds are golden brown.
3. Toss the steamed broccoli with the almond mixture.
4. Serve immediately.

Nutrition Info (per serving):

- Calories: 100 Protein: 4g Carbohydrates: 9g Dietary Fiber: 4g Sugars: 2g
- Fat: 7g Saturated Fat: 1g Sodium: 15mg

Serves: 4

Cooking Time: 10 minutes

11. Sweet Potato Fries

Ingredients:

- 2 large sweet potatoes, peeled and cut into thin strips
- 2 tablespoons olive oil
- 1 teaspoon paprika
- 1 teaspoon garlic powder

Instructions:

1. Preheat the oven to 425°F (220°C).
2. In a large bowl, toss the sweet potato strips with olive oil, paprika, and garlic powder.
3. Spread the sweet potatoes in a single layer on a baking sheet.
4. Bake for 25-30 minutes, turning halfway through, until crispy and golden brown.
5. Serve immediately.

Nutrition Info (per serving):

- Calories: 150
- Protein: 2g
- Carbohydrates: 24g
- Dietary Fiber: 4g
- Sugars: 6g
- Fat: 6g
- Saturated Fat: 1g
- Sodium: 20mg

Serves: 4

Cooking Time: 30 minutes

12. Garlic Spinach Sauté

Ingredients:

- 4 cups fresh spinach leaves
- 2 tablespoons olive oil
- 3 cloves garlic, minced
- 1 teaspoon crushed red pepper flakes

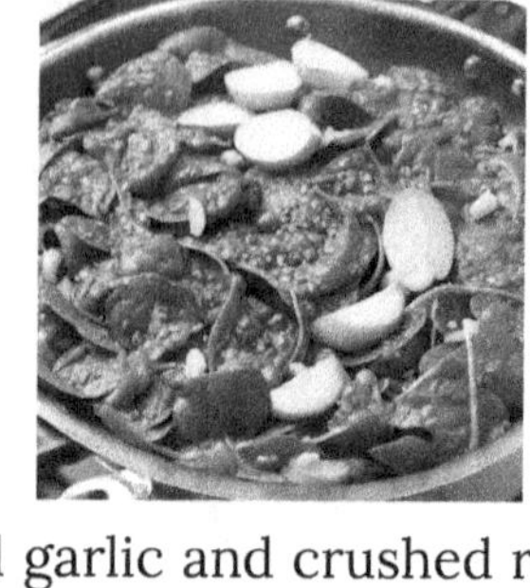

Instructions:

1. In a large skillet, heat olive oil over medium heat. Add garlic and crushed red pepper flakes, and sauté for 1-2 minutes until fragrant.
2. Add spinach leaves and sauté until wilted, about 3-4 minutes.
3. Serve immediately.

Nutrition Info (per serving):

- Calories: 100 Protein: 2g Carbohydrates: 5g Dietary Fiber: 2g Sugars: 0g
- Fat: 9g Saturated Fat: 1.5g
- Sodium: 50mg

Serves: 4

Cooking Time: 10 minutes

13. Tomato Basil Bruschetta

Ingredients:

- 4 Roma tomatoes, diced
- 1/4 cup chopped fresh basil
- 2 cloves garlic, minced
- 1 tablespoon olive oil
- 1 tablespoon balsamic vinegar
- 1 baguette, sliced

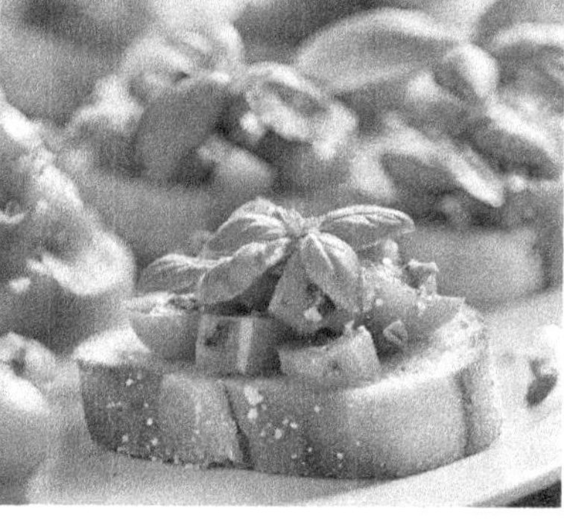

Instructions:

1. Preheat the oven to 400°F (200°C).
2. In a medium bowl, combine diced tomatoes, basil, garlic, olive oil, and balsamic vinegar.
3. Arrange baguette slices on a baking sheet and toast in the oven for 5-7 minutes until lightly browned.
4. Spoon the tomato mixture onto each toasted baguette slice.
5. Serve immediately.

Nutrition Info (per serving):

- Calories: 150 Protein: 4g Carbohydrates: 20g Dietary Fiber: 2g Sugars: 3g
- Fat: 6g
- Saturated Fat: 1g
- Sodium: 150mg

Serves: 4

Cooking Time: 15 minutes

14. Zucchini Noodles with Pesto

Ingredients:

- 4 medium zucchinis, spiralized
- 1/2 cup basil pesto (store-bought or homemade)
- 1 tablespoon olive oil
- 1/4 cup grated Parmesan cheese

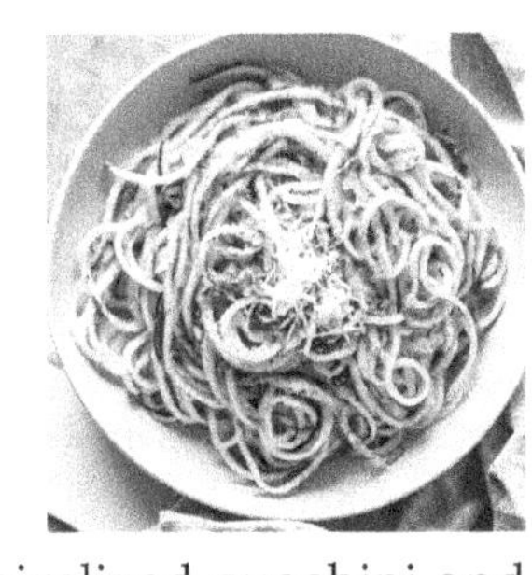

Instructions:

1. In a large skillet, heat olive oil over medium heat. Add spiralized zucchini and sauté for 3-4 minutes until tender.
2. Remove from heat and toss with basil pesto.
3. Sprinkle with grated Parmesan cheese before serving.
4. Serve immediately.

Nutrition Info (per serving):

- Calories: 140 Protein: 4g Carbohydrates: 8g Dietary Fiber: 2g Sugars: 5g
- Fat: 11g Saturated Fat: 2g Sodium: 150mg

Serves: 4

Cooking Time: 10 minutes

15. Baked Apples with Cinnamon

Ingredients:

- 4 large apples, cored and sliced
- 2 tablespoons maple syrup
- 1 teaspoon ground cinnamon
- 1/4 cup chopped walnuts

Instructions:

1. Preheat the oven to 375°F (190°C).
2. In a large bowl, toss apple slices with maple syrup and ground cinnamon.
3. Arrange the apples in a baking dish and sprinkle with chopped walnuts.
4. Bake for 25-30 minutes until the apples are tender.
5. Serve warm.

Nutrition Info (per serving):

- Calories: 150
- Protein: 2g
- Carbohydrates: 28g
- Dietary Fiber: 5g
- Sugars: 22g
- Fat: 5g
- Saturated Fat: 0.5g
- Sodium: 2mg

Serves: 4

Cooking Time: 30 minutes

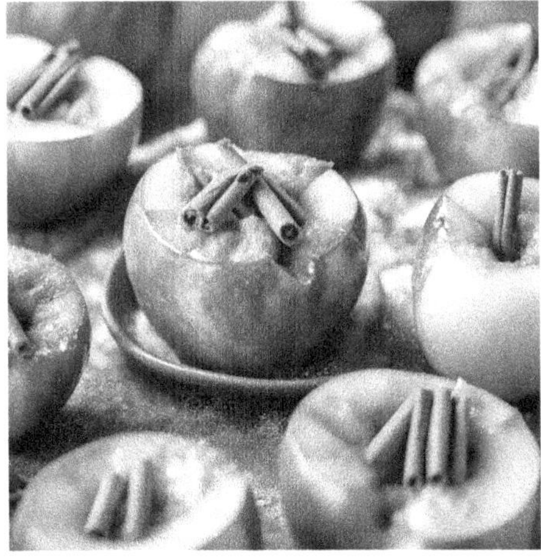

16. Frozen Yogurt Bark

Ingredients:

- 2 cups plain Greek yogurt
- 2 tablespoons honey
- 1/2 cup mixed berries (blueberries, strawberries, raspberries)
- 1/4 cup chopped nuts (almonds, walnuts)

Instructions:

1. Line a baking sheet with parchment paper.
2. In a bowl, mix together Greek yogurt and honey.
3. Spread the yogurt mixture evenly on the prepared baking sheet.
4. Sprinkle mixed berries and chopped nuts on top.
5. Freeze for 2-3 hours until firm.
6. Break into pieces and serve.

Nutrition Info (per serving):

- Calories: 120
- Protein: 8g
- Carbohydrates: 12g
- Dietary Fiber: 2g
- Sugars: 10g
- Fat: 4g
- Saturated Fat: 0.5g
- Sodium: 35mg

Serves: 4

Cooking Time: 3 hours (freezing time)

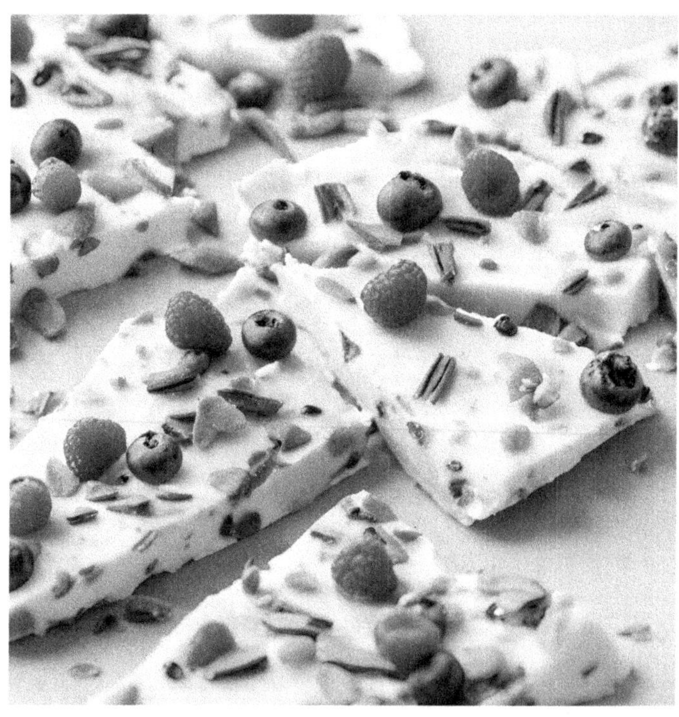

17. Baba Ganoush

Ingredients:

- 1 large eggplant
- 2 tablespoons tahini
- 2 cloves garlic, minced
- 1/4 cup lemon juice
- 1 tablespoon olive oil
- 1/2 teaspoon ground cumin

Instructions:

1. Preheat the oven to 400°F (200°C).
2. Prick the eggplant several times with a fork and place it on a baking sheet.
3. Roast the eggplant for 35-40 minutes until the skin is charred and the flesh is soft.
4. Let the eggplant cool, then scoop out the flesh and place it in a food processor.
5. Add tahini, garlic, lemon juice, olive oil, and cumin to the food processor and blend until smooth.
6. Serve with pita bread or vegetable sticks.

Nutrition Info (per serving):

- Calories: 90
- Protein: 2g
- Carbohydrates: 10g
- Dietary Fiber: 4g
- Sugars: 4g
- Fat: 5g
- Saturated Fat: 0.5g
- Sodium: 10mg

Serves: 4

Cooking Time: 40 minutes

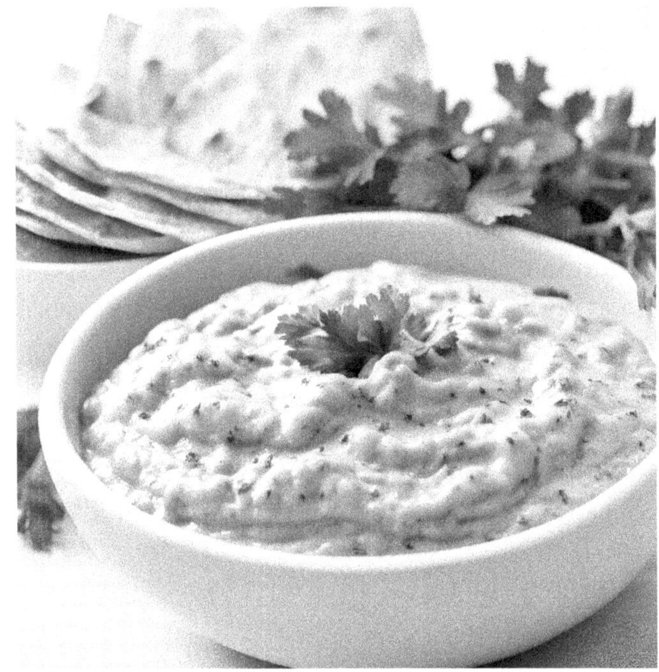

18. Red Pepper Hummus

Ingredients:

- 1 can (15 oz) chickpeas, drained and rinsed
- 1 red bell pepper, roasted and peeled
- 2 tablespoons tahini
- 2 cloves garlic, minced
- 1/4 cup lemon juice
- 1 tablespoon olive oil
- 1/2 teaspoon smoked paprika

Instructions:

1. In a food processor, combine chickpeas, roasted red bell pepper, tahini, garlic, lemon juice, olive oil, and smoked paprika.
2. Blend until smooth and creamy.
3. Serve with pita bread or vegetable sticks.

Nutrition Info (per serving):

- Calories: 100 Protein: 4g Carbohydrates: 12g Dietary Fiber: 4g Sugars: 2g
- Fat: 5g Saturated Fat: 0.5g Sodium: 120mg

Serves: 4

Cooking Time: 10 minutes

19. Black Bean Dip

Ingredients:

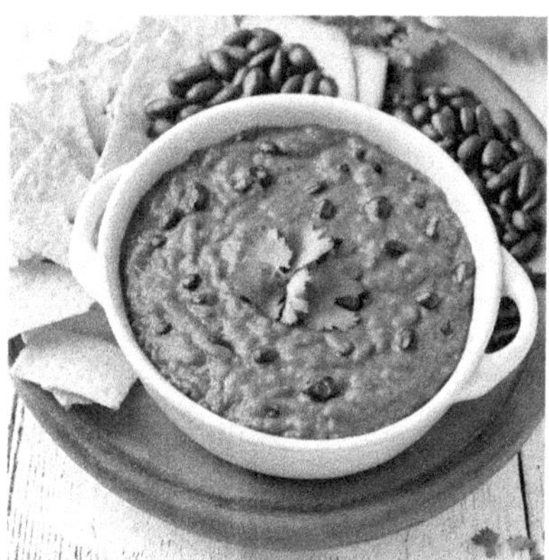

- 1 can (15 oz) black beans, drained and rinsed
- 1/4 cup salsa
- 2 tablespoons lime juice
- 1 clove garlic, minced
- 1 teaspoon ground cumin
- 1/4 cup chopped fresh cilantro

Instructions:

1. In a food processor, combine black beans, salsa, lime juice, garlic, and cumin.
2. Blend until smooth.
3. Stir in chopped cilantro.
4. Serve with tortilla chips or vegetable sticks.

Nutrition Info (per serving):

- Calories: 80 Protein: 4g Carbohydrates: 15g Dietary Fiber: 6g Sugars: 1g
- Fat: 1g
- Saturated Fat: 0g
- Sodium: 200mg

Serves: 4

Cooking Time: 10 minutes

20. Antioxidant Salad

Ingredients:

- 4 cups mixed salad greens
- 1 cup fresh blueberries
- 1 cup fresh strawberries, sliced
- 1/2 cup pomegranate seeds
- 1/4 cup chopped walnuts
- 1/4 cup crumbled feta cheese
- 2 tablespoons balsamic vinegar
- 1 tablespoon olive oil

Instructions:

1. In a large bowl, combine salad greens, blueberries, strawberries, pomegranate seeds, walnuts, and feta cheese.
2. In a small bowl, whisk together balsamic vinegar and olive oil.
3. Drizzle the dressing over the salad and toss gently to combine.
4. Serve immediately.

Nutrition Info (per serving):

- Calories: 150
- Protein: 4g
- Carbohydrates: 20g
- Dietary Fiber: 5g
- Sugars: 12g
- Fat: 8g
- Saturated Fat: 2g
- Sodium: 100mg

Serves: 4

Cooking Time: 10 minutes

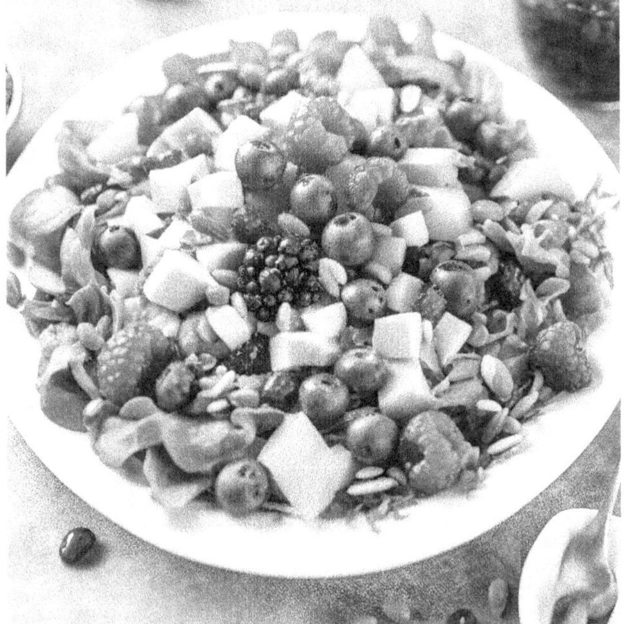

Desserts Recipes

1. Grilled Peaches with Cinnamon
Ingredients:
- 4 large peaches, halved and pitted
- 2 tablespoons honey
- 1 teaspoon ground cinnamon

Instructions:
1. Preheat the grill to medium-high heat.
2. Brush the cut sides of the peaches with honey.
3. Sprinkle ground cinnamon over the honey-coated peaches.
4. Place the peaches on the grill, cut side down.
5. Grill for 3-4 minutes until the peaches are tender and have grill marks.
6. Serve warm.

Nutrition Info (per serving):
- Calories: 100 Protein: 1g Carbohydrates: 25g Dietary Fiber: 3g Sugars: 22g
- Fat: 0g
- Saturated Fat: 0g
- Sodium: 0mg

Serves: 4
Cooking Time: 10 minutes

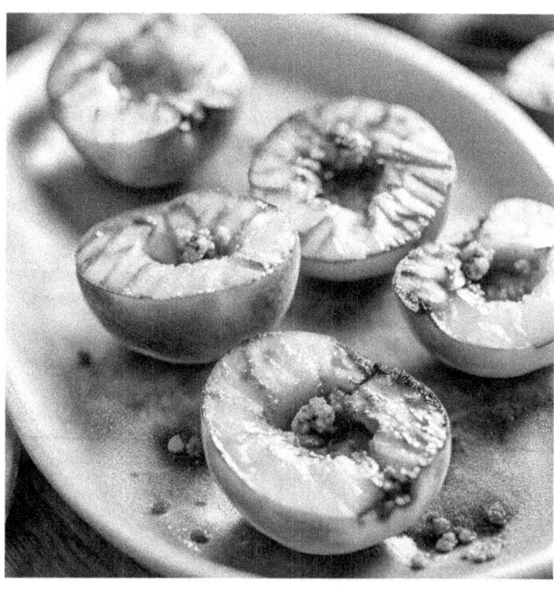

2. Berry Compote with Vanilla Yogurt

Ingredients:

- 2 cups mixed berries (blueberries, strawberries, raspberries)
- 2 tablespoons honey
- 1 teaspoon lemon juice
- 1 teaspoon vanilla extract
- 2 cups vanilla Greek yogurt

Instructions:

1. In a medium saucepan, combine mixed berries, honey, and lemon juice.
2. Cook over medium heat for 5-7 minutes until the berries are soft and the mixture thickens.
3. Remove from heat and stir in vanilla extract.
4. Let the berry compote cool to room temperature.
5. Divide the vanilla yogurt into four bowls and top with the berry compote.
6. Serve immediately.

Nutrition Info (per serving):

- Calories: 140 Protein: 8g Carbohydrates: 25g Dietary Fiber: 4g Sugars: 20g
- Fat: 2g Saturated Fat: 1g Sodium: 40mg

Serves: 4

Cooking Time: 10 minutes

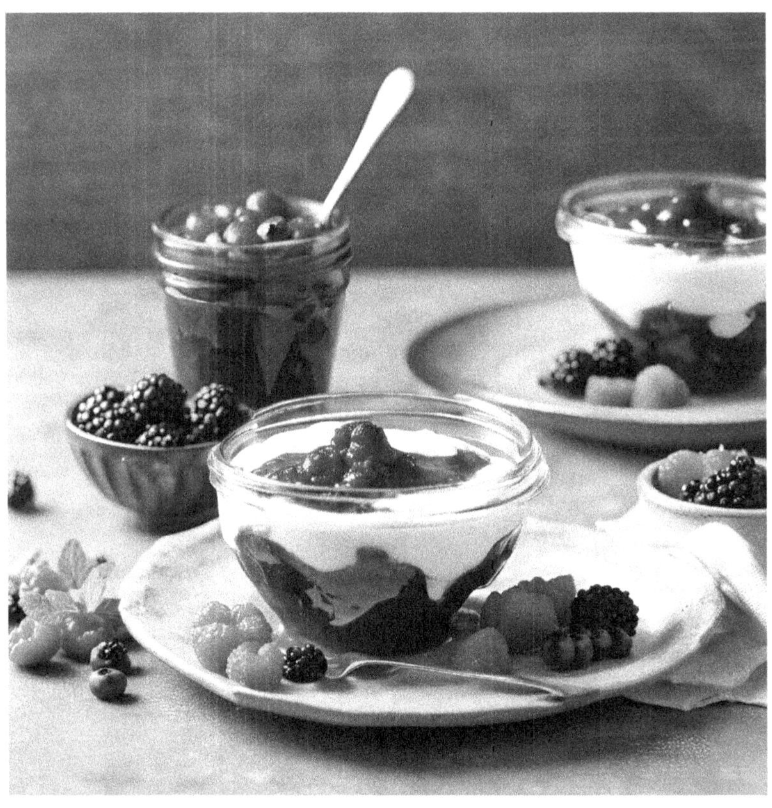

3. Baked Apples with Nutmeg and Cloves

Ingredients:

- 4 large apples, cored
- 2 tablespoons honey
- 1 teaspoon ground nutmeg
- 1/2 teaspoon ground cloves
- 1/4 cup chopped walnuts

Instructions:

1. Preheat the oven to 375°F (190°C).
2. Place the apples in a baking dish.
3. Drizzle honey over the apples.
4. Sprinkle ground nutmeg and cloves over the honey-coated apples.
5. Fill the center of each apple with chopped walnuts.
6. Bake for 25-30 minutes until the apples are tender.
7. Serve warm.

Nutrition Info (per serving):

- Calories: 150
- Protein: 2g
- Carbohydrates: 28g
- Dietary Fiber: 5g
- Sugars: 22g
- Fat: 5g
- Saturated Fat: 0.5g
- Sodium: 1mg

Serves: 4

Cooking Time: 30 minutes

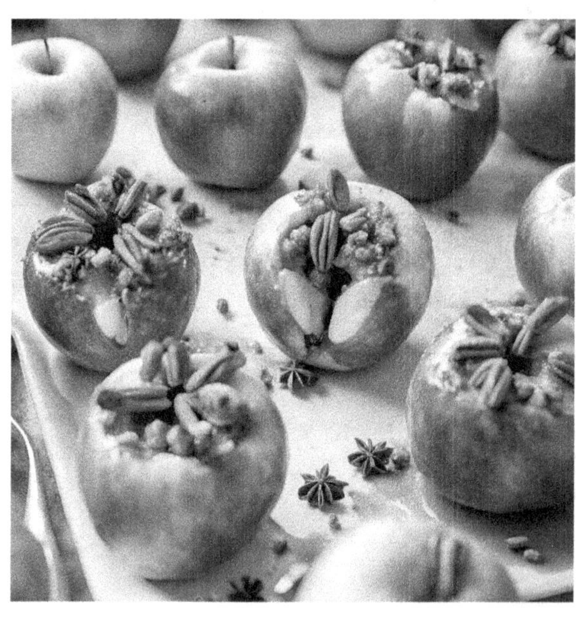

4. Papaya Boats

Ingredients:

- 2 ripe papayas, halved and seeded
- 1 cup Greek yogurt
- 1/2 cup granola
- 1/4 cup honey
- 1/4 cup mixed berries (blueberries, strawberries, raspberries)

Instructions:

1. Scoop out some of the papaya flesh to create a larger cavity.
2. Fill each papaya half with Greek yogurt.
3. Top with granola, honey, and mixed berries.
4. Serve immediately.

Nutrition Info (per serving):

- Calories: 220 Protein: 6g Carbohydrates: 40g Dietary Fiber: 5g Sugars: 30g
- Fat: 5g Saturated Fat: 1g
- Sodium: 35mg

Serves: 4

Cooking Time: 10 minutes

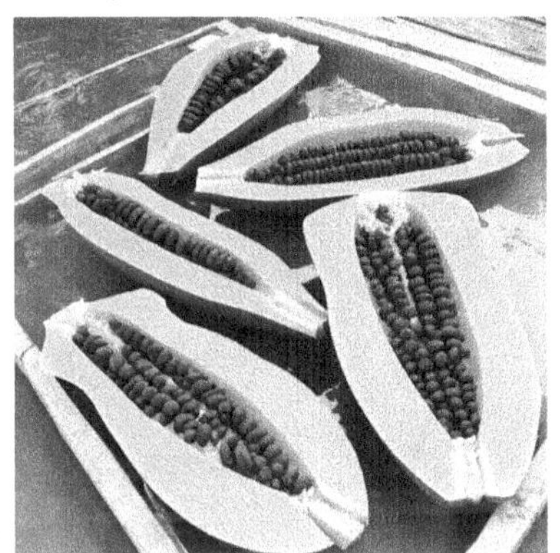

5. Kiwi and Pineapple Parfait

Ingredients:

- 2 cups Greek yogurt
- 1 cup fresh pineapple, diced
- 2 kiwis, peeled and sliced
- 1/4 cup granola
- 2 tablespoons honey

Instructions:

1. In four serving glasses, layer Greek yogurt, pineapple, and kiwi slices.
2. Sprinkle granola on top of each parfait.
3. Drizzle honey over the granola.
4. Serve immediately.

Nutrition Info (per serving):

- Calories: 180
- Protein: 8g
- Carbohydrates: 32g
- Dietary Fiber: 3g
- Sugars: 25g
- Fat: 3g
- Saturated Fat: 1g
- Sodium: 40mg

Serves: 4

Cooking Time: 10 minutes

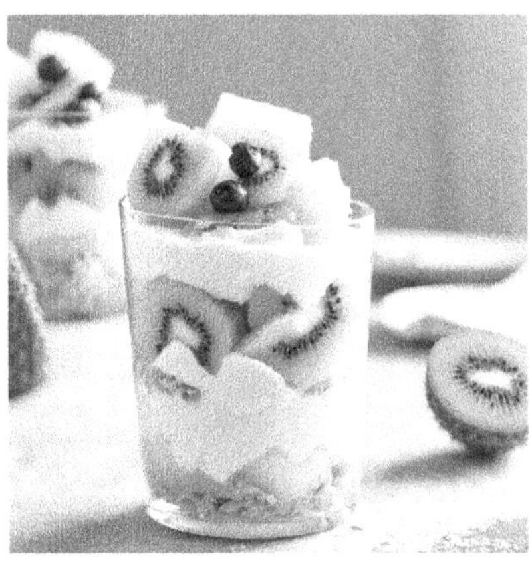

6. Apple Pear Crisp

Ingredients:

- 2 large apples, peeled and sliced
- 2 large pears, peeled and sliced
- 1/4 cup rolled oats
- 1/4 cup whole wheat flour
- 1/4 cup brown sugar
- 1/4 cup chopped walnuts
- 2 tablespoons coconut oil, melted
- 1 teaspoon ground cinnamon

Instructions:

1. Preheat the oven to 350°F (175°C).
2. In a large bowl, combine apples and pears. Spread them evenly in a baking dish.
3. In another bowl, mix together rolled oats, whole wheat flour, brown sugar, chopped walnuts, coconut oil, and ground cinnamon.
4. Sprinkle the oat mixture evenly over the fruit.
5. Bake for 25-30 minutes until the topping is golden brown and the fruit is tender.
6. Serve warm.

Nutrition Info (per serving):

- Calories: 220
- Protein: 3g
- Carbohydrates: 38g
- Dietary Fiber: 5g
- Sugars: 24g
- Fat: 8g
- Saturated Fat: 3g
- Sodium: 15mg

Serves: 4
Cooking Time: 30 minutes

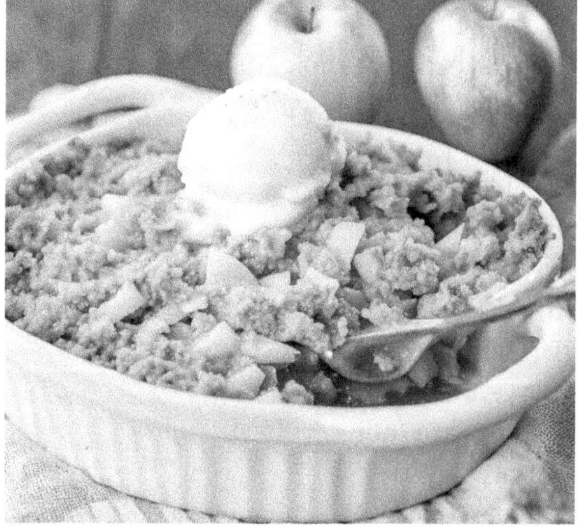

7. Chia Pudding with Almond Milk

Ingredients:

- 1/4 cup chia seeds
- 1 cup unsweetened almond milk
- 1 tablespoon honey
- 1/2 teaspoon vanilla extract
- 1/4 cup fresh berries (optional)

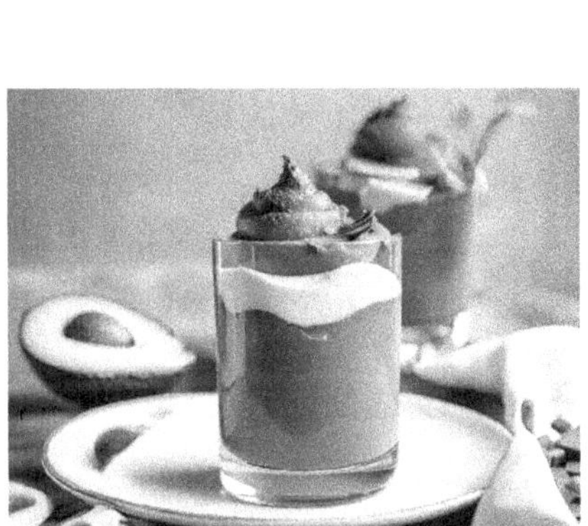

Instructions:

1. In a bowl, mix together chia seeds, almond milk, honey, and vanilla extract.
2. Cover and refrigerate for at least 4 hours, or overnight, until the mixture thickens.
3. Stir the pudding and divide into serving bowls.
4. Top with fresh berries if desired.
5. Serve chilled.

Nutrition Info (per serving):

- Calories: 150 Protein: 4g Carbohydrates: 16g Dietary Fiber: 7g Sugars: 10g
- Fat: 8g Saturated Fat: 0.5g Sodium: 50mg

Serves: 2

Cooking Time: 4 hours (refrigeration time)

8. Avocado Chocolate Mousse

Ingredients:

- 2 ripe avocados
- 1/4 cup unsweetened cocoa powder
- 1/4 cup honey
- 1 teaspoon vanilla extract
- 1/4 cup almond milk

Instructions:

1. In a blender or food processor, combine avocados, cocoa powder, honey, vanilla extract, and almond milk.
2. Blend until smooth and creamy.
3. Divide the mousse into serving bowls and refrigerate for at least 1 hour before serving.

Nutrition Info (per serving):

- Calories: 200 Protein: 2g Carbohydrates: 30g Dietary Fiber: 7g Sugars: 18g
- Fat: 12g
- Saturated Fat: 2g
- Sodium: 20mg

Serves: 4

Cooking Time: 10 minutes (plus 1 hour refrigeration)

9. Pumpkin Custard

Ingredients:

- 1 can (15 oz) pumpkin puree
- 1 cup unsweetened almond milk
- 2 eggs
- 1/4 cup maple syrup
- 1 teaspoon ground cinnamon
- 1/2 teaspoon ground nutmeg
- 1/2 teaspoon ground ginger

Instructions:

1. Preheat the oven to 350°F (175°C).
2. In a large bowl, whisk together pumpkin puree, almond milk, eggs, maple syrup, cinnamon, nutmeg, and ginger.
3. Pour the mixture into a baking dish.
4. Bake for 45-50 minutes, until the custard is set and a knife inserted into the center comes out clean.
5. Allow to cool before serving.

Nutrition Info (per serving):

- Calories: 130
- Protein: 4g
- Carbohydrates: 20g
- Dietary Fiber: 2g
- Sugars: 12g
- Fat: 4g
- Saturated Fat: 1g
- Sodium: 30mg

Serves: 6

Cooking Time: 50 minutes

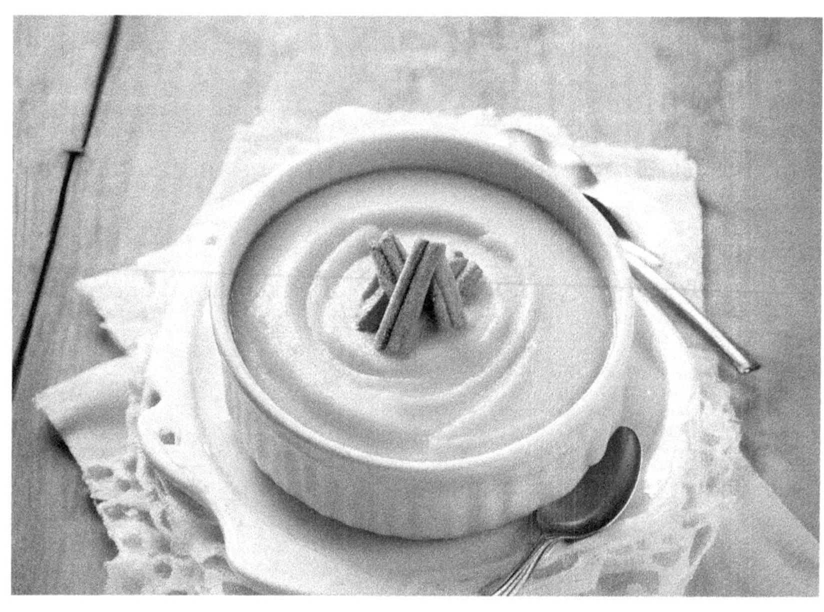

10. Almond Flour Carrot Cake

Ingredients:

- 2 cups almond flour
- 1 cup grated carrots
- 1/4 cup honey
- 3 eggs
- 1/4 cup coconut oil, melted
- 1 teaspoon vanilla extract
- 1 teaspoon ground cinnamon
- 1/2 teaspoon baking soda
- 1/4 teaspoon ground nutmeg

Instructions:

1. Preheat the oven to 350°F (175°C). Grease an 8-inch round cake pan.
2. In a large bowl, mix together almond flour, cinnamon, baking soda, and nutmeg.
3. In another bowl, whisk together eggs, honey, coconut oil, and vanilla extract.
4. Stir the wet ingredients into the dry ingredients until well combined.
5. Fold in the grated carrots.
6. Pour the batter into the prepared cake pan and spread evenly.
7. Bake for 25-30 minutes, until a toothpick inserted into the center comes out clean.
8. Allow the cake to cool before serving.

Nutrition Info (per serving):

- Calories: 220
- Protein: 6g
- Carbohydrates: 15g
- Dietary Fiber: 4g
- Sugars: 10g
- Fat: 16g
- Saturated Fat: 6g
- Sodium: 100mg

Serves: 8

Cooking Time: 30 minutes

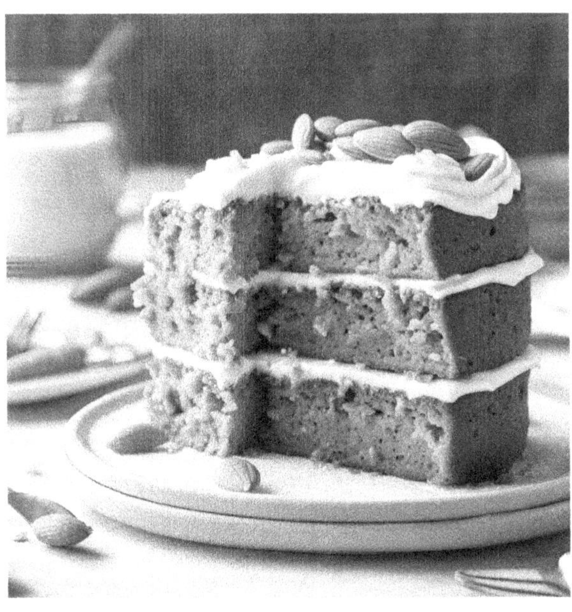

11. Banana Oat Muffins

Ingredients:

- 2 ripe bananas, mashed
- 1 cup rolled oats
- 1/2 cup almond flour
- 2 eggs
- 1/4 cup honey
- 1 teaspoon vanilla extract
- 1 teaspoon baking powder
- 1/2 teaspoon ground cinnamon

Instructions:

1. Preheat the oven to 350°F (175°C) and line a muffin tin with paper liners.
2. In a large bowl, mix together mashed bananas, rolled oats, almond flour, baking powder, and cinnamon.
3. In another bowl, whisk together eggs, honey, and vanilla extract.
4. Stir the wet ingredients into the dry ingredients until well combined.
5. Divide the batter evenly among the muffin cups.
6. Bake for 20-25 minutes, until a toothpick inserted into the center comes out clean.
7. Allow to cool before serving.

Nutrition Info (per serving):

- Calories: 120
- Protein: 4g
- Carbohydrates: 20g
- Dietary Fiber: 3g
- Sugars: 8g
- Fat: 4g
- Saturated Fat: 0.5g
- Sodium: 70mg

Serves: 12

Cooking Time: 25 minutes

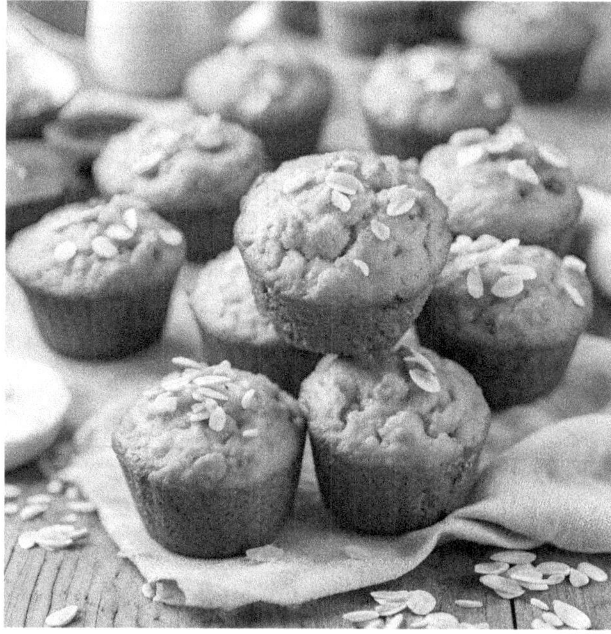

12. Pumpkin Bars

Ingredients:

- 1 cup pumpkin puree
- 1/2 cup almond butter
- 1/4 cup honey
- 2 eggs
- 1 teaspoon vanilla extract
- 1/2 cup almond flour
- 1 teaspoon ground cinnamon
- 1/2 teaspoon ground nutmeg
- 1/2 teaspoon baking soda

Instructions:

1. Preheat the oven to 350°F (175°C) and grease a 9x9-inch baking pan.
2. In a large bowl, mix together pumpkin puree, almond butter, honey, eggs, and vanilla extract until smooth.
3. Stir in almond flour, cinnamon, nutmeg, and baking soda until well combined.
4. Pour the batter into the prepared pan and spread evenly.
5. Bake for 20-25 minutes, until a toothpick inserted into the center comes out clean.
6. Allow to cool before cutting into bars and serving.

Nutrition Info (per serving):

- Calories: 130
- Protein: 4g
- Carbohydrates: 15g
- Dietary Fiber: 2g
- Sugars: 10g
- Fat: 7g
- Saturated Fat: 1g
- Sodium: 70mg

Serves: 9

Cooking Time: 25 minutes

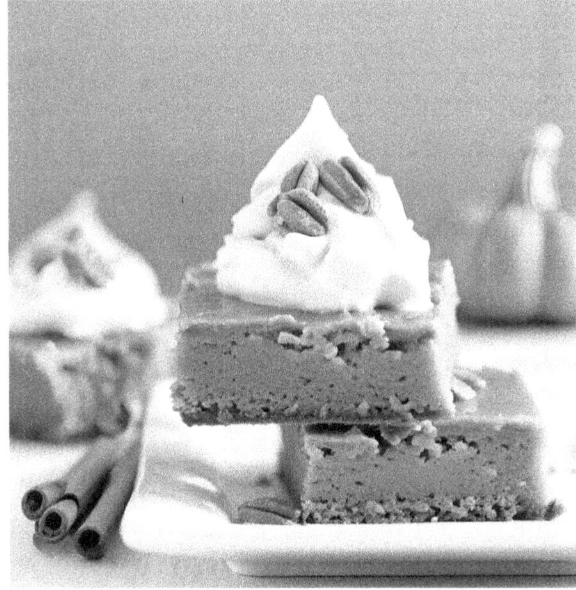

13. Sweet Potato Brownies

Ingredients:

- 1 cup mashed sweet potatoes
- 1/2 cup almond butter
- 1/4 cup cocoa powder
- 1/4 cup honey
- 1 teaspoon vanilla extract
- 2 eggs
- 1/2 teaspoon baking soda

Instructions:

1. Preheat the oven to 350°F (175°C) and grease an 8x8-inch baking pan.
2. In a large bowl, mix together mashed sweet potatoes, almond butter, cocoa powder, honey, vanilla extract, eggs, and baking soda until smooth.
3. Pour the batter into the prepared pan and spread evenly.
4. Bake for 20-25 minutes, until a toothpick inserted into the center comes out clean.
5. Allow to cool before cutting into squares and serving.

Nutrition Info (per serving):

- Calories: 140
- Protein: 4g
- Carbohydrates: 18g
- Dietary Fiber: 3g
- Sugars: 10g
- Fat: 7g
- Saturated Fat: 1g
- Sodium: 70mg

Serves: 9

Cooking Time: 25 minutes

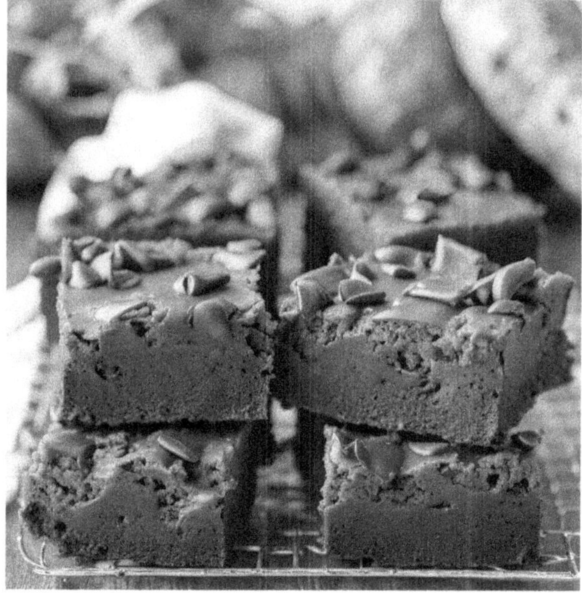

14. Strawberry Lemonade Popsicles

Ingredients:

- 2 cups fresh strawberries, hulled
- 1 cup lemon juice
- 1/2 cup water
- 1/4 cup honey

Instructions:

1. In a blender, combine strawberries, lemon juice, water, and honey.
2. Blend until smooth.
3. Pour the mixture into popsicle molds.
4. Freeze for at least 4 hours until solid.
5. Serve frozen.

Nutrition Info (per serving):

- Calories: 60   Protein: 0.5g   Carbohydrates: 16g   Dietary Fiber: 1g   Sugars: 14g
- Fat: 0g
- Saturated Fat: 0g
- Sodium: 1mg

Serves: 6

Cooking Time: 4 hours (freezing time)

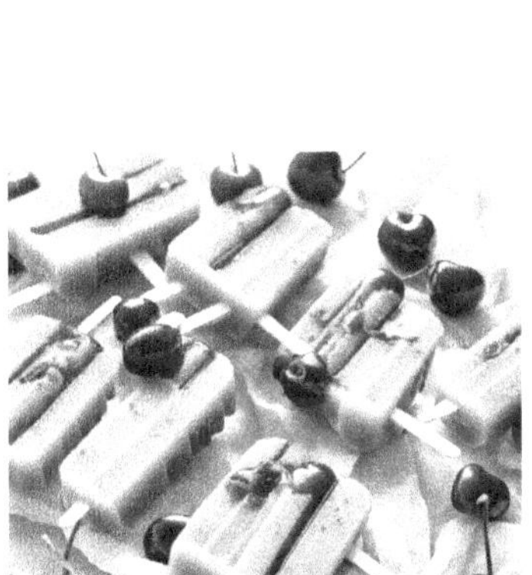

15. Cherry Almond Ice Pops

Ingredients:

- 2 cups fresh cherries, pitted
- 1 cup unsweetened almond milk
- 1/4 cup honey
- 1 teaspoon almond extract

Instructions:

1. In a blender, combine cherries, almond milk, honey, and almond extract.
2. Blend until smooth.
3. Pour the mixture into popsicle molds.
4. Freeze for at least 4 hours until solid.
5. Serve frozen.

Nutrition Info (per serving):

- Calories: 70   Protein: 1g   Carbohydrates: 17g   Dietary Fiber: 1g
- Sugars: 14g
- Fat: 0.5g
- Saturated Fat: 0g
- Sodium: 5mg

Serves: 6

Cooking Time: 4 hours (freezing time)

16. Pineapple Carpaccio

Ingredients:

- 1 pineapple, peeled and thinly sliced
- 1 tablespoon honey
- 1 tablespoon lime juice
- 1/4 cup fresh mint leaves, chopped

Instructions:

1. Arrange the pineapple slices on a large serving platter.
2. In a small bowl, mix together honey and lime juice
. 3. Drizzle the honey-lime mixture over the pineapple slices.
1. Sprinkle with chopped mint leaves.
2. Serve immediately.

Nutrition Info (per serving):

- Calories: 80
- Protein: 1g
- Carbohydrates: 20g
- Dietary Fiber: 2g
- Sugars: 17g
- Fat: 0g
- Saturated Fat: 0g
- Sodium: 1mg

Serves: 4

Cooking Time: 10 minutes

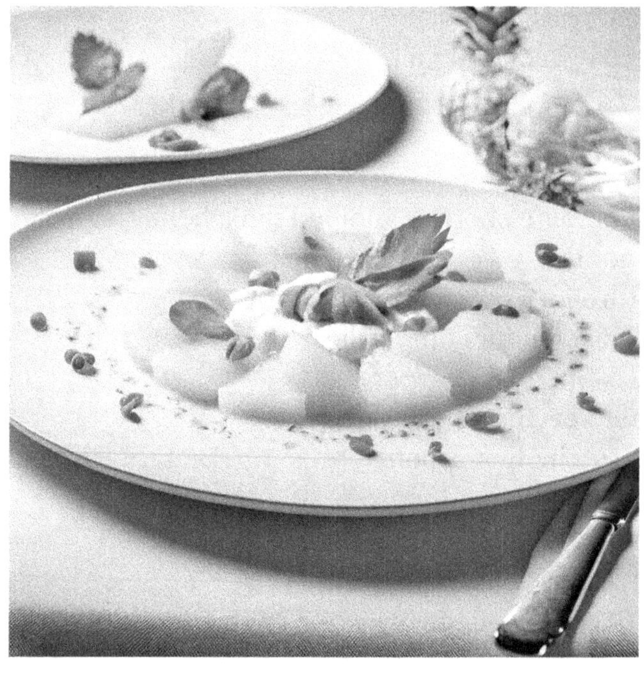

17. Grapefruit Brûlée

Ingredients:

- 2 large grapefruits, halved
- 2 tablespoons honey
- 1 teaspoon ground cinnamon

Instructions:

1. Preheat the broiler to high.
2. Place the grapefruit halves on a baking sheet.
3. Drizzle each grapefruit half with honey.
4. Sprinkle ground cinnamon over the honey.
5. Broil for 3-5 minutes until the tops are caramelized.
6. Serve warm.

Nutrition Info (per serving):

- Calories: 60 Protein: 1g   Carbohydrates: 15g Dietary Fiber: 2g Sugars: 13g
- Fat: 0g Saturated Fat: 0g
- Sodium: 0mg

Serves: 4

Cooking Time: 5 minutes

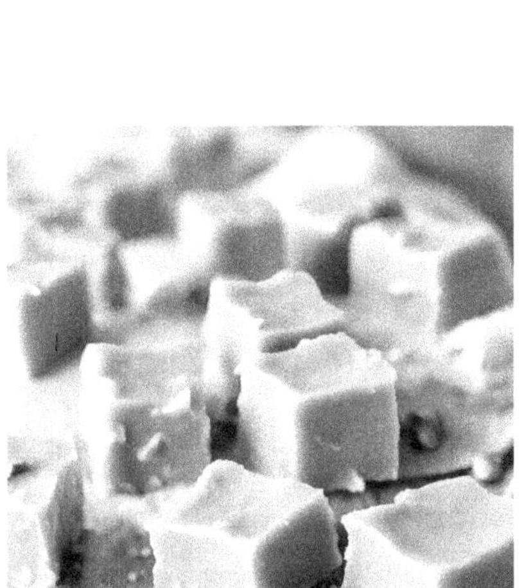

18. Cashew Vanilla Fudge

Ingredients:

- 1 cup raw cashews
- 1/4 cup coconut oil, melted
- 1/4 cup honey
- 1 teaspoon vanilla extract
- 1/4 teaspoon ground cinnamon

Instructions:

1. In a food processor, blend raw cashews until smooth and creamy.
2. Add melted coconut oil, honey, vanilla extract, and ground cinnamon. Blend until well combined.
3. Line a small baking dish with parchment paper and pour the mixture into the dish.
4. Freeze for at least 1 hour until firm.
5. Cut into squares and serve.

Nutrition Info (per serving):

- Calories: 120   Protein: 2g Carbohydrates: 10g Dietary Fiber: 1g Sugars: 8g
- Fat: 8g
- Saturated Fat: 4g
- Sodium: 2mg

Serves: 12

Cooking Time: 1 hour (freezing time)

19. Walnut and Date Loaf

Ingredients:

- 1 cup whole wheat flour
- 1 cup rolled oats
- 1/2 cup chopped walnuts
- 1/2 cup chopped dates
- 1/4 cup honey
- 2 eggs
- 1/2 cup unsweetened almond milk
- 1 teaspoon baking soda
- 1 teaspoon ground cinnamon

Instructions:

1. Preheat the oven to 350°F (175°C) and grease a loaf pan.
2. In a large bowl, mix together whole wheat flour, rolled oats, baking soda, and ground cinnamon.
3. In another bowl, whisk together eggs, honey, and almond milk.
4. Stir the wet ingredients into the dry ingredients until well combined.
5. Fold in chopped walnuts and dates.
6. Pour the batter into the prepared loaf pan and spread evenly.
7. Bake for 40-45 minutes, until a toothpick inserted into the center comes out clean.
8. Allow to cool before slicing and serving.

Nutrition Info (per serving):

- Calories: 180
- Protein: 4g
- Carbohydrates: 30g
- Dietary Fiber: 3g
- Sugars: 12g
- Fat: 6g
- Saturated Fat: 1g
- Sodium: 120mg

Serves: 10

Cooking Time: 45 minutes

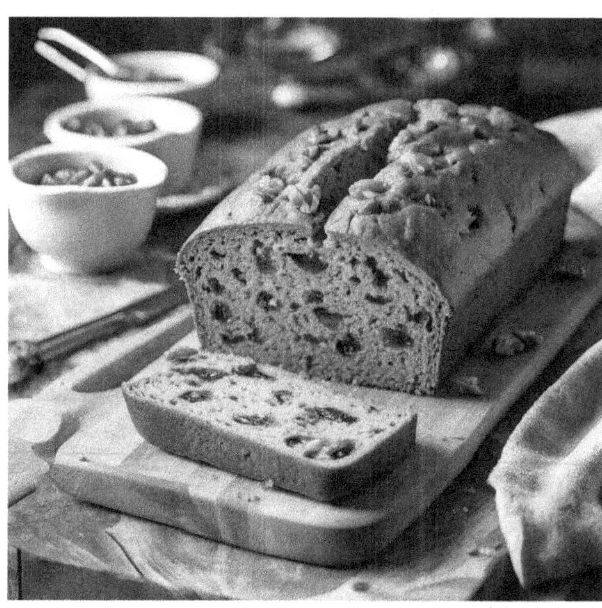

10-WEEK MEAL PLAN

Week 1

Day 1

- **Breakfast**: Blueberry Spinach Smoothie
- **Lunch**: Mediterranean Stuffed Chicken
- **Dinner**: Quinoa Tabbouleh with Steamed Broccoli and Almond Slivers
- **Snack**: Edamame with Sea Salt

Day 2

- **Breakfast**: Cherry Almond Smoothie
- **Lunch**: Chicken Caesar Salad
- **Dinner**: Slow Cooker Moroccan Chicken with Quinoa
- **Snack**: Carrot Sticks with Hummus

Day 3

- **Breakfast**: Oatmeal with Walnuts and Berries
- **Lunch**: Greek Lemon Chicken Skewers with a side salad
- **Dinner**: Turkey and Sweet Potato Stew
- **Snack**: Almond Yogurt with Honey and Walnuts

Day 4

- **Breakfast**: Quinoa Porridge
- **Lunch**: Smoky Paprika Chicken with Sweet Potato Fries
- **Dinner**: Chicken and Quinoa Soup
- **Snack**: Stuffed Dates with Almond Butter

Day 5

- **Breakfast**: Turmeric Scrambled Eggs with a side of berries
- **Lunch**: Chicken and Vegetable Kabobs
- **Dinner**: Herb Grilled Turkey Steaks with Garlic Spinach Sauté
- **Snack**: Berry Compote with Vanilla Yogurt

Day 6

- **Breakfast**: Sweet Potato Hash
- **Lunch**: Chicken Piccata with steamed vegetables
- **Dinner**: Spiced Roast Turkey with a side of roasted vegetables
- **Snack**: Frozen Yogurt Bark

Day 7

- **Breakfast**: Buckwheat Pancakes
- **Lunch**: Turkey Chili with a side salad
- **Dinner**: Baked Apples with Nutmeg and Cloves
- **Snack**: Avocado Chocolate Mousse

Week 2

Day 8

- **Breakfast**: Spinach and Feta Omelet
- **Lunch**: Chicken Vegetable Soup
- **Dinner**: Lemon Thyme Poached Cod with a side of roasted vegetables
- **Snack**: Baba Ganoush with vegetable sticks

Day 9

- **Breakfast**: Mushroom and Herb Frittata
- **Lunch**: Smoky Paprika Chicken with Quinoa Tabbouleh
- **Dinner**: Chicken and Mushroom Casserole
- **Snack**: Grilled Peaches with Cinnamon

Day 10

- **Breakfast**: Zucchini and Bell Pepper Mini Quiches
- **Lunch**: Turkey Spinach Meatballs with a side salad
- **Dinner**: Salmon Chowder
- **Snack**: Pineapple Carpaccio

Day 11

- **Breakfast**: Avocado Egg Bake
- **Lunch**: Turkey Stuffed Bell Peppers
- **Dinner**: Mediterranean Fish Stew
- **Snack**: Chia Pudding with Almond Milk

Day 12

- **Breakfast**: Tomato and Basil Egg Muffins
- **Lunch**: Chicken Caesar Salad
- **Dinner**: Polenta with Roasted Vegetables
- **Snack**: Grapefruit Brûlée

Day 13

- **Breakfast**: Berry Almond Breakfast Quinoa
- **Lunch**: Herb Grilled Turkey Steaks with Garlic Spinach Sauté
- **Dinner**: Steamed Halibut with Greens
- **Snack**: Strawberry Lemonade Popsicles

Day 14

- **Breakfast**: Overnight Oats with Pumpkin Seeds
- **Lunch**: Chicken and Quinoa Soup
- **Dinner**: Saffron Poached Haddock with a side of roasted vegetables
- **Snack**: Cashew Vanilla Fudge

Week 3

Day 15
- **Breakfast**: Smoked Salmon Breakfast Bowl
- **Lunch**: Mediterranean Stuffed Chicken
- **Dinner**: Chicken and Sweet Potato Bake
- **Snack**: Stuffed Dates with Almond Butter

Day 16
- **Breakfast**: Almond Butter and Banana Toast
- **Lunch**: Chicken Caesar Salad
- **Dinner**: Grilled Sardines with Lemon and Herbs
- **Snack**: Walnut and Date Loaf

Day 17
- **Breakfast**: Nutty Rice Cakes
- **Lunch**: Spiced Roast Turkey with Quinoa Tabbouleh
- **Dinner**: Steamed Broccoli with Almond Slivers and Chicken Piccata
- **Snack**: Sweet Potato Fries

Day 18
- **Breakfast**: Baked Pear with Walnuts
- **Lunch**: Turkey Chili with a side salad
- **Dinner**: Mediterranean Fish Stew
- **Snack**: Almond Yogurt with Honey and Walnuts

Day 19
- **Breakfast**: Savory Vegetable Muffins
- **Lunch**: Smoky Paprika Chicken with Quinoa Tabbouleh
- **Dinner**: Saffron Poached Haddock with a side of roasted vegetables
- **Snack**: Frozen Yogurt Bark

Day 20
- **Breakfast**: Polenta with Roasted Vegetables
- **Lunch**: Chicken and Mushroom Casserole
- **Dinner**: Salmon Chowder
- **Snack**: Grilled Peaches with Cinnamon

Day 21
- **Breakfast**: Matcha Green Tea Latte with a side of berries
- **Lunch**: Lemon Thyme Poached Cod with a side of roasted vegetables
- **Dinner**: Chicken and Sweet Potato Bake
- **Snack**: Chia Pudding with Almond Milk

Week 4

Day 22

- **Breakfast**: Kale Chips
- **Lunch**: Turkey Spinach Meatballs with a side salad
- **Dinner**: Steamed Broccoli with Almond Slivers and Herb Grilled Turkey Steaks
- **Snack**: Berry Compote with Vanilla Yogurt

Day 23

- **Breakfast**: Edamame with Sea Salt
- **Lunch**: Chicken Piccata with steamed vegetables
- **Dinner**: Spiced Roast Turkey with a side of roasted vegetables
- **Snack**: Baked Apples with Nutmeg and Cloves

Day 24

- **Breakfast**: Almond Yogurt with Honey and Walnuts
- **Lunch**: Chicken Vegetable Soup
- **Dinner**: Mediterranean Fish Stew
- **Snack**: Avocado Chocolate Mousse

Day 25

- **Breakfast**: Carrot Sticks with Hummus
- **Lunch**: Chicken Caesar Salad
- **Dinner**: Polenta with Roasted Vegetables
- **Snack**: Pineapple Carpaccio

Day 26

- **Breakfast**: Calcium-Fortified Orange Juice Smoothie
- **Lunch**: Smoky Paprika Chicken with Quinoa Tabbouleh
- **Dinner**: Steamed Halibut with Greens
- **Snack**: Grilled Peaches with Cinnamon

Day 27

- **Breakfast**: Oat Bran Muffins
- **Lunch**: Turkey Chili with a side salad
- **Dinner**: Chicken and Mushroom Casserole
- **Snack**: Frozen Yogurt Bark

Day 28

- **Breakfast**: Roasted Chickpeas
- **Lunch**: Lemon Thyme Poached Cod with a side of roasted vegetables
- **Dinner**: Chicken and Sweet Potato Bake
- **Snack**: Cashew Vanilla Fudge

Week 5

Day 29

- **Breakfast**: Spinach and Feta Omelet
- **Lunch**: Herb Grilled Turkey Steaks with Garlic Spinach Sauté
- **Dinner**: Slow Cooker Moroccan Chicken with Quinoa
- **Snack**: Avocado Chocolate Mousse

Day 30

- **Breakfast**: Mushroom and Herb Frittata
- **Lunch**: Chicken Caesar Salad
- **Dinner**: Saffron Poached Haddock with a side of roasted vegetables
- **Snack**: Frozen Yogurt Bark

Day 31

- **Breakfast**: Zucchini and Bell Pepper Mini Quiches
- **Lunch**: Chicken Vegetable Soup
- **Dinner**: Salmon Nicoise Salad
- **Snack**: Pineapple Carpaccio

Day 32

- **Breakfast**: Avocado Egg Bake
- **Lunch**: Smoky Paprika Chicken with Quinoa Tabbouleh
- **Dinner**: Mediterranean Fish Stew
- **Snack**: Baked Apples with Nutmeg and Cloves

Day 33

- **Breakfast**: Tomato and Basil Egg Muffins
- **Lunch**: Turkey Spinach Meatballs with a side salad
- **Dinner**: Chicken and Mushroom Casserole
- **Snack**: Chia Pudding with Almond Milk

Day 34

- **Breakfast**: Berry Almond Breakfast Quinoa
- **Lunch**: Chicken Piccata with steamed vegetables
- **Dinner**: Herb Grilled Turkey Steaks with Garlic Spinach Sauté
- **Snack**: Grilled Peaches with Cinnamon

Day 35

- **Breakfast**: Overnight Oats with Pumpkin Seeds
- **Lunch**: Chicken and Vegetable Kabobs
- **Dinner**: Steamed Halibut with Greens
- **Snack**: Edamame with Sea Salt

Week 6

Day 36

- **Breakfast**: Smoked Salmon Breakfast Bowl
- **Lunch**: Turkey Chili with a side salad
- **Dinner**: Lemon Thyme Poached Cod with a side of roasted vegetables
- **Snack**: Carrot Sticks with Hummus

Day 37

- **Breakfast**: Almond Butter and Banana Toast
- **Lunch**: Chicken Caesar Salad
- **Dinner**: Spiced Roast Turkey with a side of roasted vegetables
- **Snack**: Berry Compote with Vanilla Yogurt

Day 38

- **Breakfast**: Nutty Rice Cakes
- **Lunch**: Mediterranean Stuffed Chicken
- **Dinner**: Chicken and Sweet Potato Bake
- **Snack**: Stuffed Dates with Almond Butter

Day 39

- **Breakfast**: Baked Pear with Walnuts
- **Lunch**: Lemon Thyme Poached Cod with a side of roasted vegetables
- **Dinner**: Salmon Chowder
- **Snack**: Roasted Chickpeas

Day 40

- **Breakfast**: Savory Vegetable Muffins
- **Lunch**: Chicken and Quinoa Soup
- **Dinner**: Mediterranean Fish Stew
- **Snack**: Grilled Peaches with Cinnamon

Day 41

- **Breakfast**: Polenta with Roasted Vegetables
- **Lunch**: Chicken Caesar Salad
- **Dinner**: Steamed Halibut with Greens
- **Snack**: Frozen Yogurt Bark

Day 42

- **Breakfast**: Matcha Green Tea Latte with a side of berries
- **Lunch**: Turkey Spinach Meatballs with a side salad
- **Dinner**: Chicken and Mushroom Casserole
- **Snack**: Avocado Chocolate Mousse

Week 7

Day 43
- **Breakfast**: Kale Chips
- **Lunch**: Spiced Roast Turkey with Quinoa Tabbouleh
- **Dinner**: Chicken and Sweet Potato Bake
- **Snack**: Chia Pudding with Almond Milk

Day 44
- **Breakfast**: Edamame with Sea Salt
- **Lunch**: Chicken Piccata with steamed vegetables
- **Dinner**: Mediterranean Fish Stew
- **Snack**: Pineapple Carpaccio

Day 45
- **Breakfast**: Almond Yogurt with Honey and Walnuts
- **Lunch**: Turkey Chili with a side salad
- **Dinner**: Saffron Poached Haddock with a side of roasted vegetables
- **Snack**: Baked Apples with Nutmeg and Cloves

Day 46
- **Breakfast**: Carrot Sticks with Hummus
- **Lunch**: Smoky Paprika Chicken with Quinoa Tabbouleh
- **Dinner**: Herb Grilled Turkey Steaks with Garlic Spinach Sauté
- **Snack**: Grilled Peaches with Cinnamon

Day 47
- **Breakfast**: Calcium-Fortified Orange Juice Smoothie
- **Lunch**: Chicken Caesar Salad
- **Dinner**: Steamed Broccoli with Almond Slivers and Chicken Piccata
- **Snack**: Berry Compote with Vanilla Yogurt

Day 48
- **Breakfast**: Oat Bran Muffins
- **Lunch**: Chicken and Vegetable Kabobs
- **Dinner**: Salmon Nicoise Salad
- **Snack**: Frozen Yogurt Bark

Day 49
- **Breakfast**: Roasted Chickpeas
- **Lunch**: Chicken and Quinoa Soup
- **Dinner**: Spiced Roast Turkey with a side of roasted vegetables
- **Snack**: Edamame with Sea Salt

Week 8

Day 50

- **Breakfast**: Spinach and Feta Omelet
- **Lunch**: Smoky Paprika Chicken with Quinoa Tabbouleh
- **Dinner**: Chicken and Mushroom Casserole
- **Snack**: Chia Pudding with Almond Milk

Day 51

- **Breakfast**: Mushroom and Herb Frittata
- **Lunch**: Lemon Thyme Poached Cod with a side of roasted vegetables
- **Dinner**: Mediterranean Fish Stew
- **Snack**: Grilled Peaches with Cinnamon

Day 52

- **Breakfast**: Zucchini and Bell Pepper Mini Quiches
- **Lunch**: Turkey Chili with a side salad
- **Dinner**: Herb Grilled Turkey Steaks with Garlic Spinach Sauté
- **Snack**: Pineapple Carpaccio

Day 53

- **Breakfast**: Avocado Egg Bake
- **Lunch**: Chicken Caesar Salad
- **Dinner**: Steamed Halibut with Greens
- **Snack**: Avocado Chocolate Mousse

Day 54

- **Breakfast**: Tomato and Basil Egg Muffins
- **Lunch**: Turkey Spinach Meatballs with a side salad
- **Dinner**: Chicken and Sweet Potato Bake
- **Snack**: Stuffed Dates with Almond Butter

Day 55

- **Breakfast**: Berry Almond Breakfast Quinoa
- **Lunch**: Chicken and Vegetable Kabobs
- **Dinner**: Salmon Chowder
- **Snack**: Baked Apples with Nutmeg and Cloves

Day 56

- **Breakfast**: Overnight Oats with Pumpkin Seeds
- **Lunch**: Chicken Piccata with steamed vegetables
- **Dinner**: Spiced Roast Turkey with a side of roasted vegetables
- **Snack**: Frozen Yogurt Bark

Week 9

Day 57

- **Breakfast**: Smoked Salmon Breakfast Bowl
- **Lunch**: Mediterranean Stuffed Chicken
- **Dinner**: Chicken and Mushroom Casserole
- **Snack**: Grilled Peaches with Cinnamon

Day 58

- **Breakfast**: Almond Butter and Banana Toast
- **Lunch**: Chicken Caesar Salad
- **Dinner**: Mediterranean Fish Stew
- **Snack**: Chia Pudding with Almond Milk

Day 59

- **Breakfast**: Nutty Rice Cakes
- **Lunch**: Turkey Chili with a side salad
- **Dinner**: Steamed Broccoli with Almond Slivers and Chicken Piccata
- **Snack**: Pineapple Carpaccio

Day 60

- **Breakfast**: Baked Pear with Walnuts
- **Lunch**: Smoky Paprika Chicken with Quinoa Tabbouleh
- **Dinner**: Herb Grilled Turkey Steaks with Garlic Spinach Sauté
- **Snack**: Berry Compote with Vanilla Yogurt

Day 61

- **Breakfast**: Savory Vegetable Muffins
- **Lunch**: Chicken and Quinoa Soup
- **Dinner**: Spiced Roast Turkey with a side of roasted vegetables
- **Snack**: Frozen Yogurt Bark

Day 62

- **Breakfast**: Polenta with Roasted Vegetables
- **Lunch**: Chicken Caesar Salad
- **Dinner**: Steamed Halibut with Greens
- **Snack**: Avocado Chocolate Mousse

Day 63

- **Breakfast**: Matcha Green Tea Latte with a side of berries
- **Lunch**: Lemon Thyme Poached Cod with a side of roasted vegetables
- **Dinner**: Chicken and Sweet Potato Bake
- **Snack**: Stuffed Dates with Almond Butter

Week 10

Day 64

- **Breakfast**: Kale Chips
- **Lunch**: Mediterranean Stuffed Chicken
- **Dinner**: Chicken and Mushroom Casserole
- **Snack**: Grilled Peaches with Cinnamon

Day 65

- **Breakfast**: Edamame with Sea Salt
- **Lunch**: Turkey Spinach Meatballs with a side salad
- **Dinner**: Steamed Halibut with Greens
- **Snack**: Pineapple Carpaccio

Day 66

- **Breakfast**: Almond Yogurt with Honey and Walnuts
- **Lunch**: Chicken Caesar Salad
- **Dinner**: Salmon Chowder
- **Snack**: Chia Pudding with Almond Milk

Day 67

- **Breakfast**: Carrot Sticks with Hummus
- **Lunch**: Smoky Paprika Chicken with Quinoa Tabbouleh
- **Dinner**: Mediterranean Fish Stew
- **Snack**: Baked Apples with Nutmeg and Cloves

Day 68

- **Breakfast**: Calcium-Fortified Orange Juice Smoothie
- **Lunch**: Turkey Chili with a side salad
- **Dinner**: Herb Grilled Turkey Steaks with Garlic Spinach Sauté
- **Snack**: Frozen Yogurt Bark

Day 69

- **Breakfast**: Oat Bran Muffins
- **Lunch**: Chicken and Quinoa Soup
- **Dinner**: Spiced Roast Turkey with a side of roasted vegetables
- **Snack**: Grilled Peaches with Cinnamon

Day 70

- **Breakfast**: Roasted Chickpeas
- **Lunch**: Lemon Thyme Poached Cod with a side of roasted vegetables
- **Dinner**: Chicken and Sweet Potato Bake
- **Snack**: Stuffed Dates with Almond Butter

Day 71

- **Breakfast**: Spinach and Feta Omelet
- **Lunch**: Chicken and Vegetable Kabobs
- **Dinner**: Steamed Broccoli with Almond Slivers and Chicken Piccata
- **Snack**: Pineapple Carpaccio

WEEKLY MEAL PLANNER JOURNAL

	BREAKFAST	LUNCH	DINNER	SNACKS
MON				
TUE				
WED				
THU				
FRI				
SAT				
SUN				

What are your primary goals for following the Polymyalgia Rheumatica diet?
Write down at least three specific objectives you hope to achieve.

WEEKLY MEAL PLANNER JOURNAL

	BREAKFAST	LUNCH	DINNER	SNACKS
MON				
TUE				
WED				
THU				
FRI				
SAT				
SUN				

How do you currently feel about your diet and eating habits?
Reflect on your current dietary patterns and their impact on your health.

WEEKLY MEAL PLANNER JOURNAL

	BREAKFAST	LUNCH	DINNER	SNACKS
MON				
TUE				
WED				
THU				
FRI				
SAT				
SUN				

Which foods do you currently eat that you believe might trigger your Polymyalgia Rheumatica symptoms? List any specific foods or food groups that you suspect might be problematic.

WEEKLY MEAL PLANNER JOURNAL

	BREAKFAST	LUNCH	DINNER	SNACKS
MON				
TUE				
WED				
THU				
FRI				
SAT				
SUN				

What are your favorite healthy foods and meals? Identify nutritious foods you already enjoy that can be included in your new diet.

WEEKLY MEAL PLANNER JOURNAL

	BREAKFAST	LUNCH	DINNER	SNACKS
MON				
TUE				
WED				
THU				
FRI				
SAT				
SUN				

What challenges do you anticipate when changing your diet, and how can you overcome them? Think about potential obstacles and solutions to stick with your new eating plan.

WEEKLY MEAL PLANNER JOURNAL

	BREAKFAST	LUNCH	DINNER	SNACKS
MON				
TUE				
WED				
THU				
FRI				
SAT				
SUN				

How will you ensure you get adequate protein while following the Polymyalgia Rheumatica diet?Consider different sources of lean protein that you can include in your meals.

WEEKLY MEAL PLANNER JOURNAL

	BREAKFAST	LUNCH	DINNER	SNACKS
MON				
TUE				
WED				
THU				
FRI				
SAT				
SUN				

How often do you plan to prepare meals at home versus eating out? Determine a balance that works for you and supports your dietary goals.

WEEKLY MEAL PLANNER JOURNAL

	BREAKFAST	LUNCH	DINNER	SNACKS
MON				
TUE				
WED				
THU				
FRI				
SAT				
SUN				

What are some healthy snack options you can have on hand to avoid unhealthy choices? List nutritious snacks that can help you stay on track.

WEEKLY MEAL PLANNER JOURNAL

	BREAKFAST	LUNCH	DINNER	SNACKS
MON				
TUE				
WED				
THU				
FRI				
SAT				
SUN				

How can you involve your family or friends in your new dietary changes? Think of ways to include your support network in your diet transition.

WEEKLY MEAL PLANNER JOURNAL

	BREAKFAST	LUNCH	DINNER	SNACKS
MON				
TUE				
WED				
THU				
FRI				
SAT				
SUN				

What are some non-food-related activities that can help you manage stress and improve your well-being? Identify hobbies or practices, such as exercise, meditation, or spending time with loved ones, that can support your overall health.

WEEKLY MEAL PLANNER JOURNAL

	BREAKFAST	LUNCH	DINNER	SNACKS
MON				
TUE				
WED				
THU				
FRI				
SAT				
SUN				

What are some potential benefits you hope to experience by following the Polymyalgia Rheumatica diet? Write down specific health improvements you are looking forward to, such as reduced pain or increased energy.

Scan the QR code below to get a surprise bonus!